PRAISE FOR THE *Gluten-Free on a Shoestring* SERIES

"Nicole is a loving baker and gifted teacher; she will hold your hand as you create stunning breads. *Gluten-Free on a Shoestring Bakes Bread* offers all the romance and flavor of traditional breads, just without the gluten. You'll never miss it!"
—ZOË FRANÇOIS, AUTHOR OF *THE NEW ARTISAN BREAD IN FIVE MINUTES A DAY*

"Going gluten-free changed my life. It's great to have a go-to resource so I can enjoy the breads that I crave."
—JASON ROBERTS, INTERNATIONALLY KNOWN CELEBRITY CHEF AND COHOST, *THE CHEW*

"Hunn successfully tackles a chief complaint voiced by special-diet newbies: sticker shock. Her practical tips for shopping and cooking to save time and money are a gift to all of us who are paying too much for too little."
—*LIVING WITHOUT*

"Hunn has not only bestowed her readers with a complete cookbook . . . but she shows us how to save money, and time, on our meals. . . . It's well worth a bite."
—*SAN FRANCISCO BOOK REVIEW*

"I highly recommend this cookbook. The recipes are accessible and especially geared for people with busy lifestyles."
—*TUCSON CITIZEN*

"From locating best values to meal planning and stocking a gluten-free pantry, this provides a range of foods from 'scratch' that can fit any budget. Highly recommended!"
—*MIDWEST BOOK REVIEW*

"Even when she's telling you something you think you already know—like grow your own vegetables—Hunn adds an extra bit of information that takes the wisdom to another level."
—*EPICURIOUS.COM*

"Hunn's approach is delicious, inexpensive and easy: no mystery at all. I'm betting that, for some wheat-sensitive households, *Gluten-Free on a Shoestring* will be life-changing."
—*JANUARY*

"Hunn is clever and optimistic. As you flip through the pages, it's hard to avoid not feeling better about your gluten-free life. Plus, the recipes will inspire you to go into the kitchen with renewed energy and hope for the future. It's well worth spending money to purchase *Gluten-Free on a Shoestring*. It will pay dividends in the future."
—*GLUTEN-FREE LIVING*

Also by Nicole Hunn

Gluten-Free on a Shoestring

Gluten-Free on a Shoestring, Quick & Easy

Gluten-Free on a Shoestring Bakes Bread

NICOLE HUNN

Gluten-Free Classic Snacks

100 Recipes for the Brand-Name Treats You Love

Da Capo
LIFE
LONG

A MEMBER OF
THE PERSEUS BOOKS GROUP

Copyright © 2015 by Nicole Hunn
Photos by Jennifer May, jennifermay.com
Food styling by Erin Jeanne McDowell, erinjeannemcdowell.com

Note: The Snyder's of Hanover Pretzel Rods recipe (page 205) includes a recipe for Pretzel Rolls, which originally appeared in *Gluten-Free on a Shoestring Bakes Bread*, page 153.

Designed by Lisa Diercks, endpaperstudio.com
Set in 9 point Benton Sans

Cataloging-in-Publication data for this book is available from the Library of Congress.
First Da Capo Press edition 2015
ISBN: 978-0-7382-1781-9 (paperback)
ISBN: 978-0-7382-1782-6 (e-book)
Published by Da Capo Press
A Member of the Perseus Books Group
www.dacapopress.com

Note: The information in this book is true and complete to the best of our knowledge. This book is intended only as an informative guide for those wishing to know more about health issues. In no way is this book intended to replace, countermand, or conflict with the advice given to you by your own physician. The ultimate decision concerning care should be made between you and your doctor. We strongly recommend you follow his or her advice. Information in this book is general and is offered with no guarantees on the part of the authors or Da Capo Press. The authors and publisher disclaim all liability in connection with the use of this book.

Da Capo Press books are available at special discounts for bulk purchases in the U.S. by corporations, institutions, and other organizations. For more information, please contact the Special Markets Department at the Perseus Books Group, 2300 Chestnut Street, Suite 200, Philadelphia, PA 19103, or call (800) 810-4145, ext. 5000, or e-mail special.markets@perseusbooks.com.

10 9 8 7 6 5 4 3 2 1

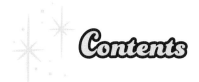

Contents

CHAPTER 3: SNACK CAKES: THE MINIATURE CAKES YOU REMEMBER — BUT BETTER *111*

Introduction

Classic Snacks (and Desserts) Are Back!

You know the old saying, you never know what you've got till it's gone? Well, I think it was written about going gluten-free. Not that I wasn't food-centric before. But being gluten-free and watching someone else mindlessly tuck in to a Drake's Coffee Cake (oh, the crumbles on top!), bite into a Kit Kat bar (break me off a piece?), or even rush off to work or school with a Quaker Oatmeal to Go square (Brown Sugar Cinnamon is my favorite) brings me to a whole other level of snack envy. Sometimes, I think I've become a woman obsessed with what used to be. And judging from the standing ovation some of these types of classic recipes have gotten when I've posted them on my blog, you're not too far behind me. If you prick us, do we not bleed? Do we, the gluten-free, not deserve all those classic snacks?

It's not that I even want to eat Entenmann's donuts every day of my life (just FYI—if I did, it would definitely be the miniature, chocolate-frosted ones). But the minute you tell me I can't have them? Well, someone's gonna pay. And I'll take that payment in cookies, crackers, and red cherry licorice, thank you. Fork over the snacks, and nobody needs to get hurt.

I have thought long and hard about why so many of us (even most of us!) love a copycat recipe for a packaged snack. I think it comes down to reliving old childhood memories and creating new memories together. And so many of the memories with family and friends that we hold most dear are created around food. Maybe you dunked Nilla Wafers in a glass of milk with your grandmother every day after school in the third grade. You don't have to leave that memory on the shelf. Or perhaps your child comes home from school, sad that everyone else seems to have Pepperidge Farm Milano cookies for lunch and she can't have them. You can give her a homemade version that's even better than the real thing. Give them all the taste of it, made with love from your own kitchen.

I do not promise that these will be the healthiest, most virtuous recipes that you make for your family. I *do*, however, promise that you will feel like Super Mom (or Dad!) when you are able to bring back Devil Dogs for your gluten-free son. And when you see your better half linger for just a few moments too long in the grocery store in front of the Mallomars, you'll feel like the best partner in the world when you serve up a spot-on homemade version the very next day. Plus, I have included recommendations wherever possible for what to use to replace some of the sugars and other ingredients in the recipes in this book with other, sometimes more healthful, ingredients. Whenever you make substitutions in a recipe, the results won't be *exactly* the same, and the treats won't taste *exactly* like the "real thing," but you decide what's best for your family!

You could, of course, survive on a steady diet of fruits, vegetables, and lean meats and maybe live a long, healthy life. But I am determined to give you the *option* of having all the treats and favorite snacks you remember so fondly. Did you have a favorite sweet while growing up? Would you love to share it with your children but you can't because, after all, your son is gluten-free and you don't want him to feel left out? Together, we can make that happen.

Most of the companies that make the original versions of these snacks are likely never going to offer a packaged gluten-free version. Some of them will (and some even do already), but we all know they will be very expensive or won't taste like the original. Or both. Plus, I can tell you from personal experience that it is just good, plain *fun* to make Kellogg's Pop-Tarts (Frosted Brown Sugar Cinnamon for me, thanks) that are a dead ringer for the original.

To get you started, I'll talk about ingredients (you didn't think I'd forget to devote a whole section to flour, did you?), tools and equipment, and tips and tricks to make your treats so much more easily. We'll begin our recipe chapters with one all about cookies. We'll cover everything from your favorite Girl Scout varieties to Nilla Wafers and Chips Ahoy! Original. Snack cakes in Chapter 3 include the likes of Little Debbie Cosmic Brownies, Hostess Sno Balls, and Tastykake Peanut Butter Kandy Kakes. Next up are crackers and other savory crunchy snacks, such as "Wheat" Thins, Ritz Bits, and crunchy pretzel rods. After that, breakfast and fruity treats are served, with everything from Kellogg's Pop-Tarts and Quaker Chewy Granola Bars to instant oatmeal flavors and Fiber One bars. Last but not least is the chapter on candy. That's where we cover licorice (both red and black), Nestlé Crunch bars, Mallo Cups, and everyone's favorite, Hershey's Kit Kat bars.

Remember, life is sweet and fun. Gluten is expendable.

With love,
Nicole

CHAPTER 1
The Basics

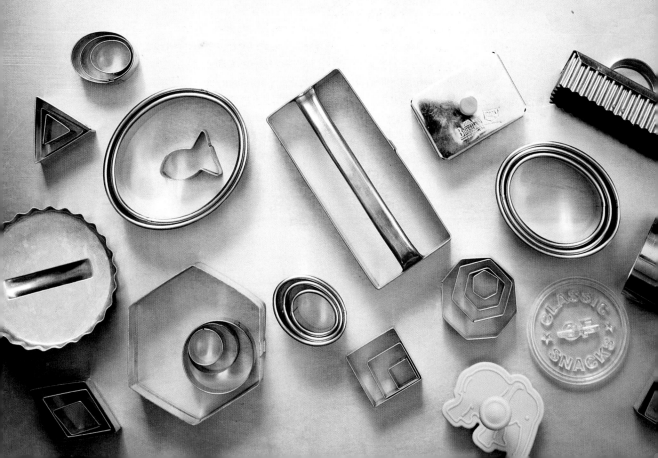

Ingredients and Substitutions

ABOUT INGREDIENTS

Many of the recipe ingredients in this book are the basic ones you will find in any baking book: butter, sugars, eggs, pure vanilla extract, baking soda, baking powder, salt, milk, and the like. However, some of the ingredients can benefit from additional explanations and details, and of course flour is its own particular concern for us, so we discuss that first. You'll also find more info on special ingredients after the flour discussion.

ABOUT SUBSTITUTIONS

Because this is a "special diet" baking book, I know that you may have questions about other allergens and ingredient substitutions. Please note that, unless I specifically state otherwise, I have *not* tested all of these recipes with the suggested substitutions. I provide these substitution suggestions based upon my extensive baking and recipe development experience. I hope they will guide you in your own experimentation if you need to make substitutions to suit your and your family's additional dietary needs. If you can't eat gluten, or need or want to eat gluten-free for any reason, every single recipe in this book will work for you when made as written. If you also have to avoid other ingredients among those in the recipes in this book, I offer you the information on pages 8–18, with love, in the hopes that your road will be made easier.

Gluten-Free Flour Blends and Components

In gluten-free baking, perhaps no issue is more important than what blend of individual gluten-free flours to use in a particular recipe, so we begin our ingredients discussion here. Because no individual gluten-free flour on its own has all the qualities of an all-purpose gluten-free flour, we must use a blend of component flours in recipes that call for an all-purpose flour. After extensive testing of commercially available, ready-made gluten-free flour blends, there are a couple that I can recommend for use in my recipes. I discuss those blends on page 3. If you must or simply prefer to blend your own all-purpose gluten-free flour, see pages 3–8, where I discuss all the potential component flours and elements, and provide recipes for the homemade flour blends that I have created and can recommend. In that section, I also list the other very simple flour blends that are necessary for some of the recipes in this book, such as a basic three-ingredient gum-free flour blend, a gluten-free cake flour, a whole-grain blend, and a bread flour blend that is used only for one recipe (Snyder's of Hanover Pretzel Rods, page 205).

If you have been baking gluten-free for some time, you have likely encountered this sort of information and are already comfortable with it. If not, this discussion may seem overwhelming, but please read it through slowly and carefully, and you'll soon find that it is mostly about providing you with options. If you want to begin simply, and in the most cost-effective way, simply purchase Better Batter Gluten Free Flour (at betterbatter.org or in retail locations where available), and use it as your all-purpose gluten-free flour.

COMMERCIALLY AVAILABLE GLUTEN-FREE FLOURS

BETTER BATTER AND CUP4CUP: After extensive testing of many of the all-purpose gluten-free flours available on the market, I have two favorite brands: Better Batter Gluten Free All Purpose Flour Mix and Cup4Cup Gluten Free Flour. Cup4Cup really works best as a pastry flour or a cake flour, as it is quite high in starch. For absolute best results for the recipes in this book, I don't recommend using it when an "all-purpose gluten-free flour" is called for, but if you do use it, the recipes will still turn out. The two homemade all-purpose gluten-free flour blend recipes that follow are the Mock Better Batter Gluten Free All Purpose Flour (page 7), which approximates the results achieved with Better Batter Gluten Free All Purpose Flour, and the Better Than Cup4Cup Gluten Free Flour, which corrects what I think is the starch imbalance in the Cup4Cup flour. Either of those blends can be used successfully in any recipe in this book that calls for an all-purpose gluten-free flour.

USING CUP4CUP AS CAKE FLOUR: If you do decide to use Cup4Cup in any recipe in this book as an "all-purpose gluten-free flour," and that recipe also calls for cornstarch, please just use more Cup4Cup, gram for gram, in place of the cornstarch. Therefore, if a recipe calls for 100 grams of all-purpose gluten-free flour and 10 grams of cornstarch, and you are using Cup4Cup as the all-purpose gluten-free flour, use 110 grams of Cup4Cup instead. Likewise, if a recipe calls for "gluten-free cake flour" and you wish to use Cup4Cup, please do not add cornstarch to the blend to create cake flour. Therefore, if a recipe calls for 100 grams of gluten-free cake flour, rather than building a gluten-free cake flour as described on page 8, just use 100 grams of Cup4Cup in place of the gluten-free cake flour.

Note: I must also caution against buying any component flours from Asian food stores, as they are often contaminated with gluten-containing grains both before reaching the store and in the store itself and may contain other additives.

HOMEMADE GLUTEN-FREE FLOUR BLENDS

GENERAL GUIDELINES: When creating your own homemade, gluten-free flour blend, you will need a simple digital kitchen scale (discussed in "Kitchen Tools and

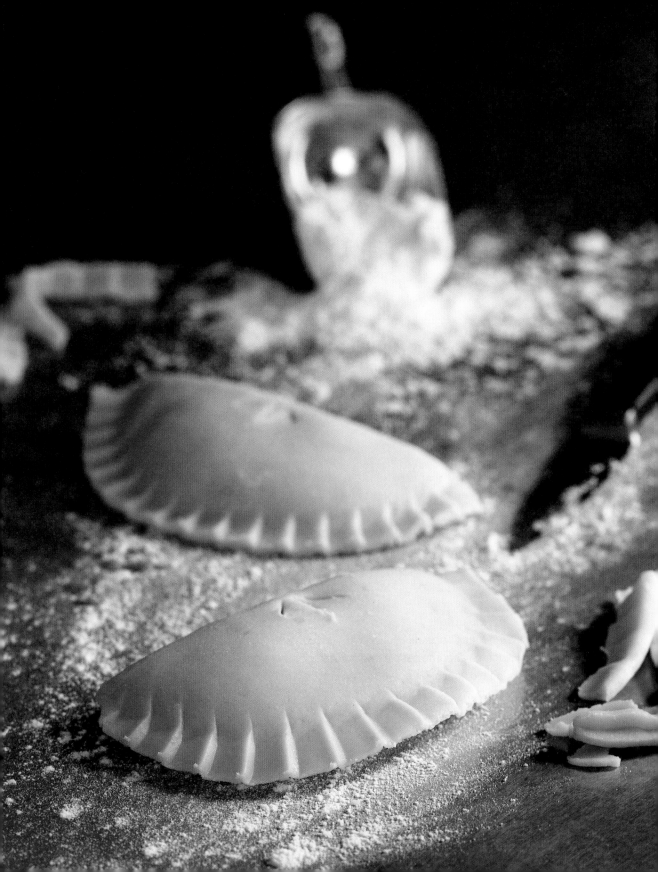

Equipment," page 20), as volume measurements are notoriously inaccurate. As discussed earlier, there is no single gluten-free flour that can serve on its own as an all-purpose gluten-free flour. In gluten-free baking, recipes developed for use with an all-purpose flour require a blend of flours to achieve the proper result. Either my Mock Better Batter Gluten Free All Purpose Flour or my Better Than Cup4Cup Gluten Free Flour recipe will work well in any recipe in this book that calls for an "all-purpose gluten-free flour."

For additional information on homemade gluten-free flour blends, please see this page on my website: http://glutenfreeonashoestring.com/all-purpose-gluten-free-flour-recipes/.

XANTHAN GUM: When a recipe calls for an "all-purpose gluten-free flour," the flour blend will already contain a specific amount of xanthan gum. (In gluten-free baking, xanthan gum helps to give batter and dough elasticity and thickness.) When a recipe calls specifically for the Basic Gum-Free Gluten-Free Flour blend, however, you'll be adding xanthan gum separately—an amount lower than would be in an all-purpose blend. Only the specific amount of xanthan gum indicated as a separate ingredient in such a recipe is appropriate. Use of an all-purpose gluten-free flour blend that already contains more xanthan gum will lead to a poor result.

MAKING MULTIPLES: All the flour blend recipes that follow can be multiplied by as many factors as you like. I typically make at least 10 cups at a time by just multiplying every ingredient by 10, placing all the ingredients in a large, airtight, lidded container, and whisking well. For an online calculator that does the math for you, please see the Flour Blends page on my website: http://glutenfreeonashoestring.com/all-purpose-gluten-free-flour-recipes/.

Each blend is as shelf-stable as each component flour is individually. Please remember that to build an all-purpose gluten-free flour successfully, you *must* use a digital kitchen scale (see page 20).

RICE FLOURS: When you're building a gluten-free flour blend, you *must* use superfine rice flours, as all other rice flours will have a gritty texture. You may not detect the grittiness of other rice flours, as some people don't, but almost everyone else will, and they will not enjoy your baked goods. They will then likely think poorly of gluten-free baked goods in general. We can't have that! The only source I know of for truly superfine rice flours is Authentic Foods. Authentic Foods superfine brown rice flour and superfine white rice flour are sold online at Authenticfoods.com and Amazon.com and also in some select brick-and-mortar stores.

POTATO FLOUR: Potato flour is made from whole potatoes that are dried and then ground into flour. It is very useful in gluten-free baking as it helps to hold baked goods together. I do not have a preference for one brand of potato flour over another. I have purchased it from Nuts.com, Authentic Foods, and Bob's Red Mill, all with similar results.

POTATO STARCH: Potato starch is made from dehydrated potatoes that have been peeled. It adds lightness to baked goods. It is a very different ingredient from potato flour. I do not have a preference for one brand of potato starch over another. I have purchased it from Nuts.com, Authentic Foods, and Bob's Red Mill, all with similar results.

TAPIOCA STARCH/FLOUR: Tapioca starch is the same thing as tapioca flour. It is very useful as it provides elasticity to gluten-free baked goods. I recommend purchasing it from either Nuts.com or Authentic Foods, companies that make a consistent-quality product. Bob's Red Mill brand tapioca starch/flour is of very inconsistent quality, as are many other brands.

PURE POWDERED FRUIT PECTIN: The powdered pectin you use must be only pure pectin, which contains no other additives (such as glucose and other sugars). I buy pectin directly from Pomona Pectin (pomonapectin.com). The pectin comes with a calcium packet; note that for the Mock Better Batter flour blend, you use only the pectin itself, not the calcium packet.

SWEET WHITE SORGHUM FLOUR: This flour is high in protein and imparts a heavier, more wheat-like texture to gluten-free baked goods. I do not have a preference for one brand of sweet white sorghum flour over another. I have purchased it from Nuts.com, Authentic Foods, and Bob's Red Mill, all with similar results.

TEFF FLOUR: Teff flour is ground from whole-grain teff (a cereal grain unrelated to wheat). It is high in protein and fiber and imparts a slightly nutty taste to gluten-free baked goods. I do not have a preference for one brand of teff flour over another. I have purchased it from Nuts.com and Bob's Red Mill with similar results.

GLUTEN-FREE BREAD FLOUR: In my bread flour blend on page 8, I buy NOW Foods unflavored whey protein isolate (which is nearly all protein—you must use isolate, not whey powder) online. For information on where to buy Expandex modified tapioca starch (including information on how to use Ultratex 3 in place of Expandex in the bread flour), please see this page on my blog, as the best place to find it often changes: http://glutenfreeonashoestring.com/gluten-free-resources/.

The Homemade Flour Blends

Remember, when building a homemade flour blend, you will achieve significantly better results when you use a simple digital kitchen scale (see page 20). I can't stress that fact enough!

———

1 cup (140 g) Mock Better Batter Gluten-Free All Purpose Flour

42 grams (about ¼ cup) superfine white rice flour (30%)

42 grams (about ¼ cup) superfine brown rice flour (30%)

21 grams (about 2⅓ tablespoons) tapioca starch/flour (15%)

21 grams (about 2⅓ teaspoons) potato starch (15%)

7 grams (about 1¾ teaspoons) potato flour (5%)

4 grams (about 2 teaspoons) xanthan gum (3%)

3 grams (about 1½ teaspoons) pure powdered fruit pectin (2%)

———

1 cup (140 g) Better Than Cup4Cup Gluten-Free Flour

42 grams (about ¼ cup) superfine white rice flour (30%)

25 grams (about 8⅓ teaspoons) cornstarch (18%)

24 grams (about 2½ tablespoons) superfine brown rice flour (17%)

21 grams (about 2⅓ tablespoons) tapioca starch/flour (15%)

21 grams (about 3⅓ tablespoons, before grinding) nonfat dry milk, ground into a finer powder (15%)

4 grams (about 1 teaspoon) potato starch (3%)

3 grams (about 1½ teaspoons) xanthan gum (2%)

———

1 cup (140 g) Basic Gum-Free Gluten-Free Flour

93 grams (about 9⅓ tablespoons) superfine white rice flour (66%)

32 grams (about 3½ tablespoons) potato starch (23%)

15 grams (about 5 teaspoons) tapioca starch/flour (11%)

———

1 cup (140 g) Gluten-Free Cake Flour

**115 grams (about 13 tablespoons) Mock Better Batter Gluten Free
All Purpose Flour (or Better Batter itself) (82%)**

25 grams (about 8⅓ teaspoons) cornstarch (18%)

1 cup (140 g) Whole-Grain Gluten-Free Flour

105 grams (about 11½ tablespoons) sweet white sorghum flour (75%)

35 grams (about ¼ cup) teff flour (25%)

1 cup (140 g) Gluten-Free Bread Flour

**100 grams (about 11½ tablespoons) Mock Better Batter Gluten Free
Flour All Purpose (or Better Batter itself) (71%)**

25 grams (about 5 tablespoons) unflavored whey protein isolate (18%)

15 grams (about 5 teaspoons) Expandex modified tapioca starch (11%)

Additional Ingredients and Substitutions

ALMOND FLOUR: The finely ground almond flour from Honeyville or Nuts.com is my preferred almond flour. Other brands are much coarser, so they perform differently in baking and tend to lead to a gritty result. If you can't have almonds, you can try substituting cashew flour or ground, raw shelled sunflower seeds in place of almond flour. If you grind the other flours yourself, they will be coarser than finely ground almond flour, so expect somewhat different results.

BUTTERMILK: The term *buttermilk* can be used to refer to the sweet liquid that is left over when cream is churned into butter. There is also "cultured" buttermilk, which is soured milk with added cultures. When you buy buttermilk in the store, it typically contains additives, such as gums and starch, which are used as thickeners. When a recipe in this book calls for buttermilk, it works best with the buttermilk that you buy at the grocery store (the kind with additives in it) because it is thicker and has a wonderful sour taste. You can also purchase and keep on hand Saco brand cultured buttermilk blend, which is a dried, powdered buttermilk. Follow the instructions on the package for how to reconstitute it. If you don't have buttermilk, though, you can "sour" nondairy or dairy milk with an acid, such as lemon juice or a mild vinegar (in a ratio of 1 cup of milk to 1 tablespoon of acid). The result won't be as thick or have quite the same flavor, but it will work in recipes that call for buttermilk.

CANOLA OIL: A few recipes in this book call for a small amount of canola oil. It is used because it is a neutral oil. Any other neutral oil, such as grapeseed oil, vegetable oil, or peanut oil, can be substituted in its place.

CERTIFIED GLUTEN-FREE OATS: Oats are not a gluten-containing grain, but unless they are "certified gluten-free," they are almost always contaminated with gluten either from being grown on or adjacent to wheat fields or stored in wheat silos. I buy certified gluten-free oats at a very reasonable price at my local Trader Joe's. The difference in varieties of oats is one of grind. From most coarse to most fine, the lineup is: oat groats, steel-cut oats, old-fashioned rolled oats, quick-cooking or instant oats, and oat flour. I don't buy all the different types. I buy one type (old-fashioned rolled oats) and pulse it in the food processor a few times for quick-cooking oats or until fine for oat flour. You can, of course, purchase the different grinds ready-made. I have never had success substituting for oats (in any grind) with any other sort of grain in my recipes, but over the years some readers have reported some success with either quinoa flakes or even gluten-free cornflake cereal.

CHOCOLATE: My favorite brand of high-quality gluten-free dark chocolate is Scharffen Berger, and I find that the best price is typically at Amazon.com. If you would like to do things the easiest way of all, purchase already-tempered chocolates of every type (milk, dark, and white, for dipping or molding) from Chocoley.com (see Resources, page 295). If you cannot have chocolate, I would recommend skipping the recipes in this book that have chocolate included in the baked good and simply eliminating the chocolate glazes and other coverings and fillings from recipes that have those.

COCOA POWDER: The recipes in the book that call for "unsweetened cocoa powder" do not specify natural cocoa powder or Dutch-processed cocoa powder. There is definitely a difference between the two in baking. Natural cocoa powder is naturally acidic and typically requires the addition of an alkaline ingredient, such as baking soda, to balance out the acidity. Dutch-processed cocoa powder is cocoa that is already alkalized to balance its acidity. It generally has a deeper, richer chocolate flavor, and I generally prefer it. But in the interest of accessibility (and cost savings), I developed and tested the recipes to accommodate either type of cocoa powder. Hershey's Special Dark unsweetened cocoa powder is a relatively economical blend of both natural and

Dutch-processed cocoa powders and works in all the recipes in this book that call for unsweetened cocoa powder. My preferred brand of Dutch-processed cocoa powder is Rodelle. It is reliably gluten-free and I buy it at Amazon.com for a relatively reasonable price. There is no substitute for cocoa powder in the recipes in this book.

CORNSTARCH: Cake flour, be it gluten-free or not, is a blend of about 80 percent all-purpose flour and about 20 percent cornstarch. It makes for a lighter baked good. Some of the recipes in this book call for "gluten-free cake flour" and others call for a certain amount of "all-purpose gluten-free flour" and another amount of "cornstarch." Please follow the recipe instructions and ingredients as written for the intended results. When a larger or smaller percentage of cornstarch is necessary, the ingredients are broken out separately. Some recipes with chocolate chips or other add-ins call for tossing the chips or other add-ins in cornstarch before adding them. This keeps the chips, or other add-ins, from sinking to the bottom of the baked good. If you can't have corn, you can try using another starch, such as potato starch or arrowroot starch, in its place in a 1:1 ratio, by weight.

EGGS: All eggs used in the recipes in this book are measured as 50 grams total (weighed out of the shell), the standard weight for large eggs. If you are using non-standard-size eggs, go by weight. If your eggs are smaller than 50 grams per egg, out of the shell, for best results beat together more than one whole egg and measure out 50 grams. I haven't tested any of these recipes with egg replacers. However, whenever I do work with an egg replacer, I have the most success by a mile with 1 chia "egg" (1 tablespoon of chia flour plus 3 tablespoons of lukewarm water), as that is the most neutral-flavored egg replacement that actually adds structure instead of just moisture. Applesauce only adds moisture, and eggs provide much more than moisture. Egg replacement, generally, will be more effective in recipes that call for a very small amount of eggs, and it will always require experimentation. For filling recipes that call for egg whites, I'm afraid that there is no substitute. Try one of the other fillings if you can't have eggs.

FLAVORING OILS: For the licorice recipes in Chapter 6, LorAnn flavoring oils are essential to achieving the intended cherry or anise flavor. LorAnn's flavoring oils are gluten-free, concentrated, and very true to the expected flavors.

GELATIN: Some of the filling recipes (see Chapter 3) and the marshmallows for the Mallomars recipe (page 65) call for powdered gelatin. I use Great Lakes unflavored gelatin, but Knox gelatin (commonly sold in 2¼-ounce packets at most grocery stores) also works perfectly well. Typically, powdered gelatin is soluble in hot water. Great

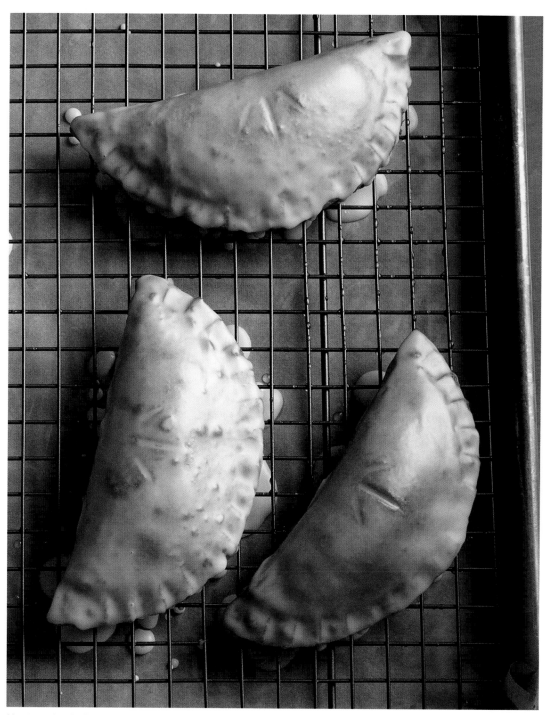

Hostess Apple Fruit Pies, page 135

Lakes also makes a cold-soluble gelatin, which does not need to be heated. It is ideal for the Stabilized Whipped Cream for Snack Cakes (page 170), as it can be used at a cool temperature, which dissolves much more easily in cold whipped cream. It is a rather specialized ingredient, however, and can be expensive. If you can use it, do so! If not, heat-soluble gelatin will work just fine. I have never worked with agar agar, which is sometimes used as a vegan substitute for powdered gelatin, but if you have experience with agar agar, give it a try!

GEL FOOD COLORINGS: For the licorice recipes in Chapter 6, gel food coloring is essential to achieving the proper intense red or black color. Liquid food coloring will not color deeply enough and will unbalance the recipe by adding too much liquid. However, if you do not like to use food coloring in anything, simply leave out the color. It does not affect the authenticity of taste.

HEAVY WHIPPING CREAM: For a non-dairy substitute for heavy whipping cream, try using the solid portion of full-fat canned coconut milk (refrigerate the can for 24 hours so the solid separates).

HONEY: There are many different flavors of honey, some much deeper and more pronounced than others. My favorite honey is wildflower, which has a relatively mild flavor. However, any honey you like can be used when it is called for in these recipes. Honey may sometimes be substituted for light corn syrup and/or Lyle's golden syrup, but it burns more easily than either of those syrups, and has a significantly more intense and recognizable flavor. So expect different results!

KOSHER SALT: I bake with kosher salt. It is considerably less concentrated than table salt, which has a significantly finer grain. It can be replaced 1:1 with lightly flaked sea salt. I find that a slightly coarse salt, such as kosher salt or lightly flaked sea salt, is much easier to use in cooking and baking than table salt, which is all too easy to accidentally overmeasure. If you would like to try substituting table salt for kosher salt in the recipes in this book, try using no more than half the volume of salt that the recipe calls for. Do not use regular sea salt, which has overly coarse grains that would not fully dissolve in your baked goods.

LIGHT CORN SYRUP: This is *not* the same as high-fructose corn syrup! Karo is the national brand that I have always used, and it is an "invert sugar," which just means that it is a mixture of two sugars (glucose and fructose) and is less likely to crystallize. It is used in candy making to prevent sugar crystals from forming. It is also used to give shine to confections and coatings, and to add sweetener without adding taste. If you can't have light corn syrup or can't find it where you live, you can replace it in the recipes in this book with Lyle's golden syrup (discussion follows) or with a rich simple syrup (see page 14). Pure glucose syrup (available at many kitchen supply stores) can also be used in place of light corn syrup.

LYLE'S GOLDEN SYRUP: Lyle's is a British sugar syrup that can be found these days in most major grocery stores in the United States. It has a distinctive, slightly toasted flavor that is quite subtle but very nice. In the recipes in this book that call for Lyle's golden syrup, if no substitute is listed in the recipe itself, you can try substituting an equal amount of Grade B maple syrup, reduced by about half in a small saucepan over low heat, or light corn syrup.

MERINGUE POWDER: Meringue powder is very useful in stabilizing buttercream frosting so that it dries stiff enough that Lofthouse Sugar Cookies (page 100) frosted with it can be stacked on top of one another without crushing the exposed frosting. LorAnn Oils brand meringue powder is gluten-free, and I have found it on Amazon.com and in larger craft and baking supply stores, both brick-and-mortar and online. Wilton states that its meringue powder has no gluten ingredients, but it cannot guarantee that the product is actually gluten-free. If you don't want to use meringue powder when it is called for in a frosting recipe or in Royal Icing (page 172), try using powdered egg whites. They tend to clump, though.

MILK: Whenever a recipe calls for milk, any kind can be used successfully, except for nonfat milk. I typically use 2% or whole dairy milk, but when I am using a nondairy milk, I much prefer unsweetened almond milk. It is richer than other types of nondairy milk, such as rice milk, and tends to be the most flavor-neutral. Whatever nondairy milk you choose, it should not be nonfat and it should be unsweetened. I have not tested the recipes in this book with nondairy milk, but it is typically one of the easiest substitutes to make in baking.

MOLASSES: Molasses is a by-product of the sugar-refining process. A few kinds of molasses are produced, but the only one called for in the recipes in this book is unsulfured molasses (the other types of molasses should not be used in its place). Most molasses sold in the United States is unsulfured, so you are likely already buying it when you buy molasses. In fact, brown sugar is simply granulated sugar with some molasses mixed into it. In place of molasses, you can try using dark corn syrup in a 1:1 ratio.

NONFAT DRY MILK: Dry milk is just what the name implies—it is simply dairy milk, evaporated into powder. I use Carnation brand. Whenever the recipes in this book include nonfat dry milk, they call for it to be ground into a finer powder. In baking, dry milk tends to remain somewhat undissolved unless it is first ground in a blender or food processor into a finer powder. There isn't a foolproof nondairy substitute for nonfat dry milk, but I have had some success using finely ground almond flour (not almond meal, which is much coarser) in its place, gram for gram, in these recipes. Some testers have had success replacing dairy nonfat dry milk with powdered coconut milk, but the only varieties of that that I have found also contain a trace amount of milk protein. If you are dairy free but that trace amount isn't a problem for you, I recommend trying powdered coconut milk in place of nonfat dry milk in the recipes in this book.

NUTELLA HAZELNUT SPREAD: The recipe for Ferrero Rocher Fine Hazelnut Chocolates (see page 281) contains Nutella hazelnut spread as an ingredient. Nutella, at least as sold in the United States, is reliably gluten-free and makes an already somewhat lengthy recipe much quicker and easier. However, if you are inclined to substitute another nut butter, it will not perform the same as Nutella, which is much thinner than other nut butters. As always, though, feel free to experiment to get it right!

OATS/OAT FLOUR: See "certified gluten-free oats," page 9.

SIMPLE SYRUP: Here is an easy substitute for light corn syrup or Lyle's Golden Syrup:
   Mix 1 cup (200 g) of granulated sugar with 1/3 cup (2 2/3 fluid ounces) of water and a pinch (1/8 teaspoon) of cream of tartar. Heat gently over low heat in a small, heavy-bottomed saucepan until all the sugar dissolves. Allow to cool completely before using. The simple syrup can be made up to a week ahead of time and stored in a sealed container in the refrigerator. It does have a tendency to crystallize over time, so longer storage is not recommended.

SOUR CREAM: Where sour cream is called for in a recipe, you can try using a nondairy sour cream or nondairy Greek-style yogurt, which should have a similar moisture content and taste to sour cream.

SPLENDA NO CALORIE SWEETENER, GRANULATED: Splenda is a brand name of sucralose, a no-calorie sugar substitute. According to the company's website, it measures 1:1 as a replacement for granulated sugar in baking, and it is stable at high temperatures, so it is suitable for baking. Splenda also makes a Splenda Sugar Blend, which is a blend of sucralose and sugar. The company states that 1/2 cup of Splenda Sugar Blend replaces 1 cup of sugar. Splenda also makes a brown sugar blend, a blend of sucralose and brown sugar, as a replacement for brown sugar in recipes. I do not care for its taste in baking, but you may like it. According to the company, Splenda is gluten-free.

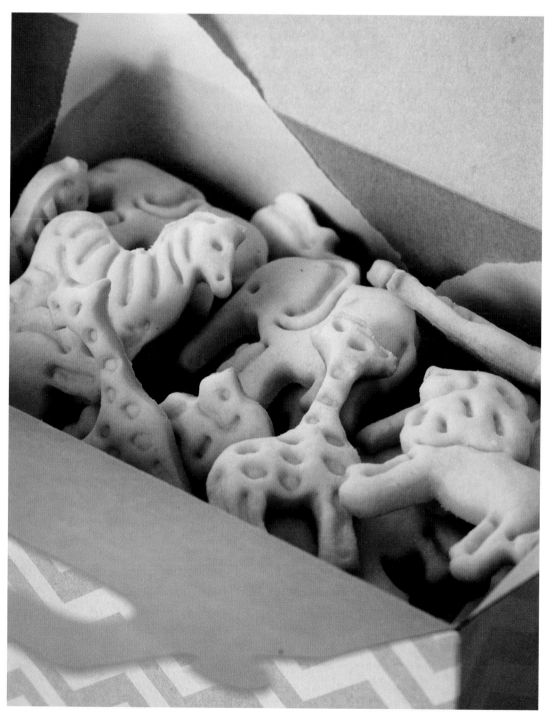

Nabisco Barnum's Animal Crackers, page 200

SUGARS: The recipes in this book call for all sorts of sugars, including granulated sugar, light brown sugar, honey, light corn syrup, molasses, Lyle's golden syrup, and confectioners' sugar. Please see the entry for each individual liquid sweetener for a thorough definition and discussion of substitutions. If you are interested in replacing any of the refined sugars in the recipes in this book with unrefined sugars and sugar-free alternatives, the recipes will not taste the same as their packaged counterparts. If you would still like to experiment, I recommend trying the following substitutions, ounce for ounce, for the nonliquid sweeteners in these recipes:

FOR CONFECTIONERS' SUGAR: Powdered Swerve (discussion follows) is the only powdered sugar substitute I am familiar with that is ground finely enough to mimic confectioners' sugar.

FOR GRANULATED SUGAR: Granulated Swerve (discussion follows), Truvia Baking Blend, or Splenda No Calorie Sweetener, Granulated.

FOR LIGHT BROWN SUGAR: Granulated coconut palm sugar, ground in a blender or food processor until finer.

SWEETENED CONDENSED MILK: For a dairy-free version of sweetened condensed milk, please visit the following page on my website: http://glutenfreeonashoestring .com/homemade-sweetened-condensed-milk/.

SWERVE: Swerve brand sweetener is a blend of erythritol (a sugar alcohol) and oligosaccharides, of which inulin (chicory root) is one. I have tried a number of sugar replacements, and Swerve is the one that I find to be the most "normal." It is not quite as sweet as cane sugar, but it is plenty sweet and it seems that the addition of inulin to the erythritol in the product cuts any "cooling" mouth feel of erythritol, which I personally find rather unpleasant in a pure erythritol sweetener. However, Swerve isn't a significant source of fiber, and doesn't come cheap. I am usually able to find it at a relatively good price on Amazon.com. Swerve also makes a powdered sugar version that dissolves well enough to make a sugar-free buttercream. To replace Swerve in the recipes that call for it, you can try using Truvia Baking Blend or Splenda. The recipes that call for Swerve (Fiber One Chewy Bars, pages 249 and 251, and VitaTops, pages 239–247) do so because I find that it behaves and tastes the most like sugar in baking, and most closely replaces the chicory root in the original, brand-name versions.

TRUVIA BAKING BLEND: Truvia is another brand-name sugar substitute. Truvia Baking Blend is a blend of erythritol, stevia leaf extract (an extract from the stevia plant), and sugar. According to the company's website, Truvia Baking Blend is preferred for baking, and it can be used to replace the sugar in a recipe at a rate of ½ cup of the baking blend to 1 cup of sugar. However, I haven't tried baking with it at all.

UNSALTED BUTTER: All the recipes in this book that include butter call for unsalted butter. Using unsalted butter in baking allows you to control the amount of salt in the recipe. If you replace the unsalted butter with salted butter, you will have to experiment with altering the salt in the recipe to compensate, as different salted butters contain different amounts of salt. As a benchmark, assume each stick of salted butter has the equivalent of about ½ teaspoon of kosher salt. If you can't have butter, I do not recommend using nondairy butter replacements, such as Earth Balance Buttery Sticks, as they have a very high moisture content. In particular, if butter replacements are used in cookies, the cookies will spread quite a lot and fail to achieve the proper consistency. You can try replacing the butter with nonhydrogenated vegetable shortening (discussion follows) in cookies, although a combination of 30 percent virgin coconut oil and 70 percent nonhydrogenated vegetable shortening would probably work best.

VEGETABLE SHORTENING: I use Spectrum Organics brand vegan nonhydrogenated vegetable shortening, both regular and butter-flavored. Crisco vegetable shortening contains hydrogenated oils, which you may prefer to avoid. Shortening has a much lower moisture content than butter, which in turn has a lower moisture content than nondairy butter substitutes, such as Earth Balance Buttery Sticks. When a recipe contains both shortening and butter, the balance is used to create the right amount of moisture to create the desired outcome in the baked good. For example, the Keebler Soft Batch Chocolate Chip Cookies (page 85) need the specific blend of butter and shortening in the recipe as written to achieve the texture, thickness, and mouthfeel of the original packaged cookies. You can certainly swap out one solid fat for another, but your results will vary. For a recipe that performs correctly and a finished baked good that tastes and looks like the original, you must follow the recipe as written. If you would like, you may successfully substitute Crisco for the nonhydrogenated vegetable shortening in any of the recipes in this book.

VIRGIN COCONUT OIL: As described more fully on pages 25–26, when making the chocolate coating or glaze for dipping cookies, snack cakes, and candies, I include virgin coconut oil in the ingredients. The oil helps to stabilize the chocolate. Therefore, you won't have to temper the chocolate to get a smooth, clean glaze that resists blooming (the white streaks that happen on melted chocolate that has hardened). Virgin coconut oil is mostly solid at room temperature and has a very mild coconut flavor. When it is melted with chocolate, it is effective as a stabilizer and the chocolate masks any coconut flavor. I buy organic virgin coconut oil for a very reasonable price at Trader Joe's, but I have seen it many places for truly outrageous prices. Shop around a bit! If you do not want or cannot have virgin coconut oil, try replacing it gram for gram with vegetable shortening (see previous discussion). Virgin coconut oil can also be an effective substitute for unsalted butter in certain recipes (see previous section on unsalted butter).

YOGURT: A few recipes call for plain yogurt. Any brand of plain yogurt will do, including nondairy soy-based and coconut-based varieties, as long as they are plain and not flavored.

Kitchen Tools and Equipment

Because this is a baking book, most of the materials you will need are fairly standard and expected, and none are particularly elaborate: whisks, large and small bowls for mixing, rimmed baking sheets (quarter and half sheet pans from Nordic Ware are my favorite), spatulas, mixing spoons, and so forth. However, there are a few additional kitchen tools and pieces of kitchen equipment that you might not expect or that can benefit from a brief explanation. These are those tools and equipment, with all the information you'll need for baking success.

CANDY/DEEP-FRY THERMOMETER: A basic candy thermometer is necessary when you make any of the candies (see Chapter 6) and fillings (see Chapter 3) in this book, as well as when you fry the Hostess Apple Fruit Pies (page 135). An analog thermometer is sufficient, and it can be a simple probe candy/deep-fry thermometer. The type of candy thermometer that tends to be easiest to use, however, is the larger, rectangular mercury candy thermometer made by Polder (and other manufacturers). It has extra metal casing at the bottom to suspend the end of the thermometer above the very end of the housing, so that you can place the thermometer on the bottom of a pot without allowing the mercury reading to be at the bottom of the pot itself. (The bottom of the pot will always be hotter than the liquid being cooked, so you need to avoid touching it with the thermometer in order to get an accurate reading.) These simple thermometers do have a tendency to lose their calibration, though, so be sure to test yours periodically by placing it in water that you bring to a boil. When the water begins to boil, the thermometer should read 212°F/100°C.

CHOCOLATE-DIPPING TOOLS: For dipping treats in melted chocolate, a standard set of dipping tools is inexpensive and will make your life a lot easier. I have a simple set of two forks (one has three tines, the other has two) and one round dipping tool for small

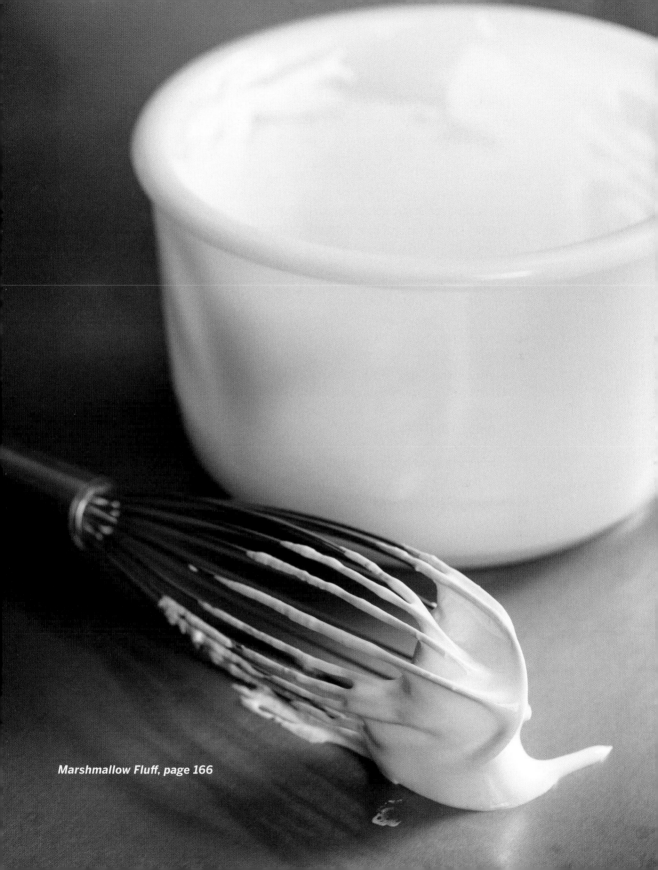

Marshmallow Fluff, page 166

round candies, such as truffles, but mostly I just use the three-tine dipping fork. Mine is made by Wilton, but Ateco also makes a very similar set. Look for a set that has tools with a handle and tines that are sturdy, so they don't bend or break during use. These sets are easy to find at Amazon.com, kitchen supply stores, and craft stores.

CHOCOLATE MOLDS: To make some of the candies from Chapter 6 in their authentic shapes, you'll need a few simple chocolate molds. A Kit Kat mold is probably the most specialized type, but it's also the most exciting type of candy to make look authentic because, c'mon—did you *ever* think you'd have a gluten-free Kit Kat? Chocolate molds are not expensive, and they're available in a number of different places online (see the Resources section, page 294). The molds you might consider purchasing are: the Kit Kat–style mold, the standard chocolate bar mold, and a mold for 100 Grand chocolate bars (each bar about 3 x 1 x ¾ inch). Of course, you can always freestyle it in a manner similar to that described in the recipe, and then cut it into whatever shapes you like.

COOKIE CUTTERS: I have way, way, way too many cookie cutters. It's an occupational hazard. But the ones I use the most, by far, are my sets of concentric circles, rectangles, squares, and ovals, both plain and scalloped. They are all made by Ateco and they come in separate, self-contained tins. I have purchased most of them at Amazon.com, but I have also found some in kitchen supply stores. I recently fell in love with spring-loaded cookie cutter/stamps. One of my favorites is the one made by Birkmann and I use it to cut out the Keebler Club Crackers (pages 176 and 177). You can find a comprehensive list of online resources that I have used for all the cookie cutters in the Resources section of this book (see page 294).

DIGITAL FOOD SCALE: There are many inexpensive digital kitchen scales on the market these days. You can find them online, at Bed Bath & Beyond, and at any kitchen supply store. All you need is a scale that can measure in both grams and ounces and is accurate to both a hundredth of an ounce and to 1 gram. I have a basic, multifunctional digital scale made by Escali (it's called the Primo and costs about $25; it has lasted for many years). The recipes in this book, and any recipes for that matter, will have by far the highest success rate when measurements are done by weight, wherever possible. This is because volume measurements from measuring cups are notoriously inaccurate. To use a digital kitchen scale, simply turn on the scale with the push of the On/Tare/Off button. Place any bowl or other container on top of the scale, "zero out" the weight of the bowl or other container by pushing "Tare" (sometimes a separate button, sometimes the same as "On/Off"), select grams (or kilograms) or ounces (or pounds), place an ingredient in the bowl until the digital counter reaches the desired weight, and then press "Tare" once more to reset to zero before adding the next ingredient. And so on . . . That's all there is to it. Once you get used to it, you'll see how much easier it makes cleanup when you no longer have to use so many different measuring cups.

DOUBLE BOILER: A classic double boiler is two nesting saucepans used to apply gentle, indirect heat to the contents of the top saucepan, which nests over the bottom saucepan. The bottom saucepan is made to hold a small amount of water, although not enough water that it touches the bottom of the top saucepan that is nesting inside of it. The bottom saucepan is placed on a stovetop and the water is brought to a simmer. It is used for sauces that require gentle heat, such as hollandaise sauce or crème anglaise. Of particular relevance here, a double boiler is also very useful for **melting chocolate**, which benefits tremendously from being heated slowly and indirectly, all but guaranteeing that it won't seize or burn. If you don't have a classic double boiler, it is very easy to jury-rig one by placing a small, heat-safe bowl on top of a small, heavy-bottomed saucepan that holds a small amount of simmering water—just make sure that the bottom of the bowl doesn't touch the surface of the water. The bowl must be big enough that its lip rests on top of the edge of the saucepan without disappearing into the saucepan. There are also so-called universal double boiler inserts that adjust to fit different size bowls, but I opt for the jury-rigged low-rent style of double boiler. It suits me. Chocolate can also easily be melted in a microwave in 30-second bursts at 60% power. For further information on tempering and melting chocolate, see page 25.

ELECTRIC MIXER: You do not *need* a stand mixer to make any of the recipes in this book. However, you will need at least a hand mixer to make a few of the recipes, such as the Marshmallow Fluff (page 166), and many of the other fillings in Chapter 2, and the marshmallows (see Mallomars, page 65). To make the Snyder's Pretzel Rods (page 205), you will need an electric mixer with dough hooks, but a five-speed hand mixer with dough hooks will work just fine. When selecting an electric hand mixer, be sure to choose a brand that sells its five-speed hand mixer with dough hooks or sells dough hooks separately that can also be purchased for use with your hand mixer. I have a KitchenAid five-speed hand mixer, which came with dough hooks, and it has performed very well over time.

GLASS STORAGE JARS: If you want your crispy cookies and especially your crackers (not to mention your Wasabi Peas, page 180) to stay crisp, store them in sealed in glass mason jars with tight-fitting lids at room temperature. If you store them in plastic, they will become soggy.

LIQUID MEASURING CUPS AND SET OF MEASURING SPOONS: Although a digital food scale (see page 20) is essential for consistent results in baking, it is typically used for dry ingredients only. Wet ingredients are still generally provided in volume measurements. However, liquid measuring cups can easily be inaccurate. To test the accuracy of your liquid measuring cup, turn on your digital kitchen scale, place the measuring cup on the scale, and press Tare to zero out the weight of the cup itself. Then, fill the cup with 1 cup (8 fluid ounces) of water by volume, and then note the weight of the water. Water is the only liquid that boasts a 1:1 equivalency between weight and volume: 1 fluid ounce of water = 1 weighted ounce of water. Since 1 cup of water = 8 fluid ounces of water, it also = 8 weighted ounces of water. If the weight of 1 cup of water by volume is not 8 weighted ounces (224 grams), your liquid measuring cup is inaccurate by the amount of the deviation. You can make allowances for that as needed. In addition, since water does have this equivalency, here are the conversions from volume to weight for water, if you would prefer to use weight for this ingredient even when volume is indicated (something I always do). Please note that these values *only* apply to water, not any other liquids:

1 cup = 8 ounces
¾ cup = 6 ounces
½ cup = 4 ounces
¼ cup = 2 ounces
2 tablespoons = 1 ounce
1 tablespoon = ½ ounce

MICROWAVE OVEN: A microwave can be very useful for small tasks, such as melting the bloomed gelatin for marshmallows (see Mallomars, page 65), melting Soft Caramel for Candies (page 291), or melting chocolate in 30-second intervals at 60% power. If you don't have a microwave, you can accomplish these small tasks by using a double boiler (see page 21).

OVEN THERMOMETER: Most ovens are off by about 50°F. Mine is off by at least that much, so I rely upon a simple oven thermometer to gauge my oven's temperature. Even if your oven is, miraculously, properly calibrated today, it may be off by next week, and if you are not using an oven thermometer, you won't know! Luckily, oven thermometers are quite inexpensive: You can find them in many places for less than $10.

PASTRY BAGS AND TIPS: You'll need a few pastry bags for filling sandwich cookies (Chapter 2), snack cakes (Chapter 3), and sandwich crackers (Chapter 4), and for decorating many of the recipes in this book. You can easily get away with using disposable bags, often without a pastry tip at all (just slice off the end of the bag to create a hole the size you want). Wilton makes disposable 12-inch pastry bags in a large roll, and they are pretty easy to find in most craft and kitchen supply stores. If 12-inch disposable pastry bags are all you can find, use them. My favorite size pastry bag is 14 inches. Not too big, not too small, it hits that sweet spot of being easy enough to handle but big enough that you can fit a fair amount of filling inside while still being able to close the top properly. If you can't close the top properly, the filling will leak right out the top of the pastry bag when you squeeze it to dispense the filling. If you can find a roll of disposable 14-inch pastry bags, grab it! If not, buy a few lined, reusable 14-inch pastry bags (Ateco makes really nice ones and they're available at nearly all craft and kitchen supply stores) and use them for all manner of filling and decoration that is white. Use disposable bags for anything with food coloring or chocolate, which may stain your reusable bag.

For pastry tips, you can buy a few individual tips or a standard set. Ateco makes really nice sets that come with their own carrying cases. The most useful tips are: Ateco or Wilton #1 and #2 for a very thin, plain line (such as on top of the Zebra Cakes, page 121), Ateco #806 or Wilton 1A tip (a nice ½-inch plain piping tip for, well, nearly everything that needs to be filled), and the Ateco or Wilton #230 (a Bismarck tip, which is a long, thin tapered piping tip with an angled edge, for piercing such snack cakes as Twinkies, page 129, and filling them).

PIZZA OR PASTRY WHEEL: To cut many of the candies in Chapter 6, the sharp blade of a pastry cutter or a pizza wheel is very handy. You can use a sharp knife instead, but rolling a cutting wheel through Soft Caramel for Candies (page 291) or Licorice (pages 287–289) is so much easier. Wilton and Ateco both make simple, effective pastry wheels, and OXO makes a great pizza wheel.

SPECIALTY SNACK CAKE PANS: I cannot stress this enough: You *do not need* any specialty snack cake pans! In each of the snack cake recipes in Chapter 3 that I made in a specialty pan, I indicate which standard baking pan can be used in its place. If you are inclined to buy any of the specialty snack cake pans, each relevant recipe indicates which manufacturers make the pans.

UNBLEACHED PARCHMENT PAPER: Unbleached parchment paper is thinner and more flexible than the bleached kind. It is essential for rolling out certain doughs, and it is the perfect nonstick surface for lining baking sheets. It can even be reused if the food you bake on it doesn't leave too much residue behind. I buy If You Care brand, and I find it at my local grocery store. However, the best price is usually at Amazon.com.

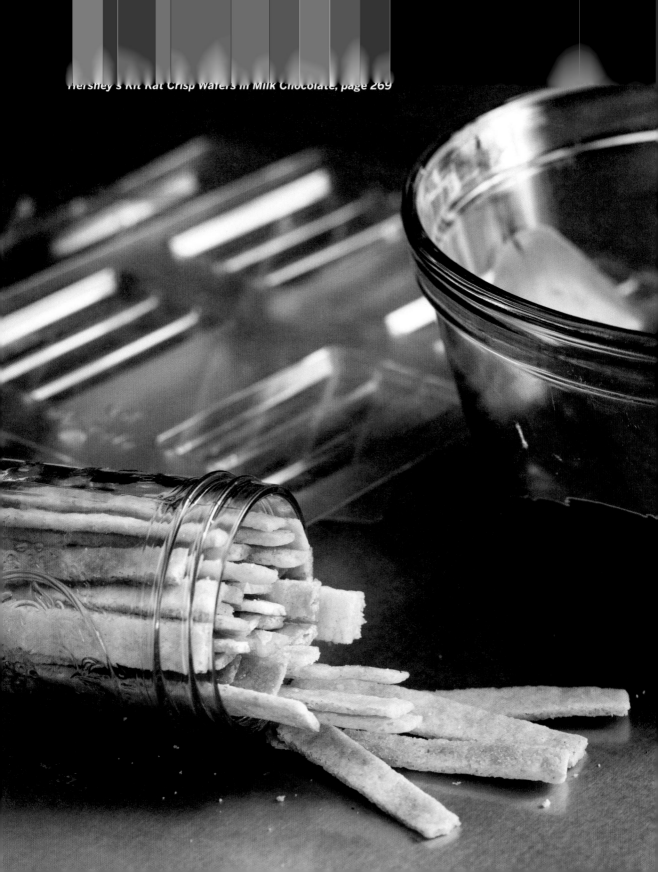

Hershey's Kit Kat Crisp Wafers in Milk Chocolate, page 269

Tips and Tricks to Make These Treats

Most of the techniques applied to the recipes in this book are pretty ordinary. Nothing too tricky here. But there are a few tasks that may be new and/or kind of intimidating. I intend to leave no man behind in this, our quest to take every imaginable classic brand-name snack and dessert—and make it gluten-free at home, anytime. These tricks and tips will help.

WORKING WITH CHOCOLATE

Different recipes throughout this book call for melted chocolate, but the way you melt it depends on how the chocolate is to be used and on your intended result.

Tempering chocolate simply means melting it in a special way that encourages the cocoa butter in the chocolate to crystallize in a particular internal pattern. When you are melting chocolate for dipping and molding, as you are for some of the recipes in this book, particularly those in Chapter 6 (Candy), it must be tempered for a few reasons. Tempered chocolate is shiny and doesn't form the white streaks, called bloom, that make it look unattractive and almost spoiled (bloom on chocolate is not a sign of spoilage, however). Tempered chocolate used for molding will also pop right out of molds very easily, unlike untempered chocolate, which tends to become grainy and stick to molds. Finally, as tempering raises the melting point of chocolate, it won't melt as easily in your hands as untempered chocolate.

When you are **melting chocolate** to bake right into a cake or cookie, there is no need to temper it. Just melt it slowly over a double boiler (directions follow) or in 30-second intervals in the microwave at about 60% power, stirring between intervals, without particular regard to temperature (just don't heat it too high, too fast or it will seize). Let the melted chocolate cool if needed and proceed with the recipe.

When you are using melted chocolate to make a glaze or a chocolate drizzle, you need a stable melted chocolate to create a smooth, clean glaze that resists blooming. Typically, the recipes in this book that require a chocolate glaze consist of chocolate melted with virgin coconut oil. This stabilizes the chocolate *without* having to temper it. The result will not be quite as stable as properly tempered chocolate, but for our at-home purposes it works perfectly well. If you are willing to temper the chocolate you are working with, however, simply eliminate the virgin coconut oil called for in the recipe, replace it with the same amount of additional chopped chocolate, by weight, and proceed with the simple tempering process that follows.

If you are on the fence about whether to properly temper chocolate, I suggest tempering it for the chocolate-covered candy recipes in Chapter 6. It is in those recipes where chocolate really takes center stage, and properly tempered chocolate for molding and dipping will result in chocolate candies that last quite well.

A simple tempering process requires a double boiler, a candy/deep-fry thermometer, and chopped chocolate (not chips!). Here are the simple steps:

1. In a medium-size, heat-safe bowl, place about three quarters of the chopped chocolate you intend to temper. Place the bowl of chocolate over a double boiler, and, using a candy/deep-fry thermometer, bring the chocolate up to 115°F, stirring gently and occasionally as it heats. Remove the chocolate from the heat and place it on a flat, heat-safe surface.

2. Stirring the chocolate gently with a spatula, add the remaining one quarter of the chopped chocolate, and continue to stir gently until the temperature of the chocolate lowers to about 88°F (in any event, below 91°F). Your chocolate is now tempered and ready for dipping or molding.

3. If the chocolate begins to set before you are done using it, warm it again over a double boiler, but don't allow it to exceed 91°F. If the temperature of the chocolate does, in fact, rise above 91°F, all is not lost. You will simply have to repeat these tempering steps and add a few more pieces of chocolate in step 2.

Dipping chocolate: If the recipe instructions call for immersing a treat in chocolate to cover it on all sides, melt the chocolate in a deep bowl with high sides. That will create a deeper pool of melted chocolate to dip in, which will make for a smoother end result. If you are at all concerned about your technique, try using even more chocolate than the recipe directs. That will allow you to truly immerse the cookie or candy in the melted chocolate by dunking it. Then, pull out the treat with a dipping fork (or the tines of a large fork) and drag it along the side of the bowl of chocolate to remove any excess. This will help avoid the "foot" that dipped chocolate can sometimes have when it isn't dipped properly. Place the chocolate-covered treat on a piece of waxed or parchment paper on a flat surface, and pull out the fork quickly.

COOKING SUGAR

A few recipes in this book call for cooking sugar, mostly to make candy (Chapter 6), but also to make some of the cookie and snack cake fillings (Chapters 2 and 3). Rest assured, these recipes don't call for any fancy techniques, and slightly imperfect results are perfectly fine.

Here are a few easy tricks that will help you achieve success when cooking sugar.

1. **Low and slow.** When cooking sugar on the stovetop, do *not* become impatient and raise the flame too high in an attempt to increase the temperature more quickly. You will likely burn the sugar and have to scrap it and begin again with fresh sugar. Cooking sugar is definitely a case of "the long way is the short way." Keep the heat at whatever level the recipe directs.

2. **Use the right size saucepan.** If you use a saucepan that is too small, the sugar

may bubble up and out of the pan. Too large and it will burn, as the mixture will be exposed to too much of the surface area of the hot pan and raise in temperature too quickly. Ideally, the initial mixture will come up at least one-third of the way up the sides of the pan and no more than halfway.

3. **Pay attention.** When cooking sugar, always use a candy/deep-fry thermometer (see page 18), and watch it carefully. The temperature tends to rise slowly, and then it can seem to jump up when you're not looking. If you exceed the proper stage, the sugar will change irrevocably. You'll have to begin again!

4. **Brush the sides.** When you first begin cooking the sugar, if it splatters against the sides of the saucepan, use a wet pastry brush to push the splatters back down into the mixture. That way, the splattered sugar won't burn.

5. **No scraping!** When you pour the cooked sugar mixture out of the pan, don't scrape the bottom. No matter how careful you were in cooking the sugar, there still may be burned bits on the bottom and it's best to leave them behind.

6. **Easy cleanup.** Cleanup from cooking sugar can seem like a big mess, but it's easy. Water is very effective at dissolving cooked sugar. Simply fill the used pot with warm water and allow it to sit. The water will break up the sugar and it should come off easily. If it doesn't, add a solution of 1 part vinegar to 3 parts water to the saucepan, making sure the liquid goes as high in the saucepan as did the sugar you are trying to clean. Place the saucepan on the stovetop over medium heat, bring it to a boil, and maintain the boil until the sugar looks like it has begun to dissolve. You should be able to remove the pot from the stove and clean it easily now.

ROLLING OUT COOKIE DOUGH AND CRACKER DOUGH

Many of the cookies in Chapter 3 belong to the category of drop cookies, which simply means the dough is portioned with a spoon or ice-cream scoop and dropped onto the prepared baking sheet for baking. Some others are slice-and-bake cookies, which are rolled into a cylinder, wrapped in parchment, and chilled before slicing by cross-section. Slice-and-bake cylinders of dough often flatten on the bottom as they chill. To correct that, either rock the cylinder back and forth as if it were a rolling pin on the counter before slicing, to round any edges, or simply slice the cookies and remold them into a round shape with your hands before baking.

Many others are so-called cut-out cookies, meaning that they are formed by rolling out the dough with a rolling pin before using a cookie cutter or knife to cut out shapes for baking. Are you less than confident about your ability to make cut-out crackers and cookies? Do you turn the page whenever you see that recipe instructions direct you to roll out cookie or cracker dough? Well, cutouts are in your future. I can *feel* it. You just won't want to miss out on all the Girl Scout Cookies (pages 34–48) and let's not forget about Mallomars (page 65) and all the Keebler crackers (pages 174–177)! Here are some tricks that will help you become more comfortable with this process:

1. **Follow the instructions** in each recipe carefully. Some will instruct you to roll out dough between two sheets of unbleached parchment paper. Others will instruct you to sprinkle a flat surface lightly with flour and sprinkle the dough lightly with flour as you roll it out. The instructions reflect what works best based upon a whole lot of trial and error and a base knowledge of which doughs can tolerate absorbing more flour and which cannot. The same holds true for how thick the dough should be rolled out. If you roll dough too thin and then bake as directed, your cookies or crackers are likely to get too crisp and perhaps burn. If you roll it too thick, the final product will not crisp as you expect. For the results you seek, follow the instructions!

2. **Feel it.** Rolling the dough out into an even layer tends to be the most challenging aspect of making cut-out cookies and crackers. The secret is much more in how it *feels* than in how it *looks*. Your hands are much more sensitive than your eyes in this regard, because your eyes really can't compare the relative thickness of the dough from one spot to another. But your hands can feel it rather well. Trust them! Run an open palm lightly over the surface of the dough (if you are rolling it out between two sheets of unbleached parchment paper, do this without removing the top sheet of parchment). Does it feel as if it's thicker in some places, thinner in others? Correct that with your rolling pin.

3. **Use the right paper.** Bleached parchment paper is thick and rather stiff. It's not an appropriate substitute for unbleached parchment paper, which is much thinner and more flexible. You will not be able to feel the dough through bleached parchment paper enough to roll it out evenly between two sheets of paper (see trick #2).

4. **Take it easy!** When rolling out dough between sheets of parchment paper, do not press too hard. If you find that you are rolling lots of creases and wrinkles into the dough, you're likely pressing too hard with the rolling pin, which is wrinkling the paper and then pressing those wrinkles into the dough. Apply less pressure with the rolling pin, and roll out stiffer doughs effectively by passing over the surface more times.

5. **Chill it!** If your dough seems difficult to cut out with clean lines or if it is sticking to the parchment paper or your hands, try wrapping it up in plastic wrap and placing it in the refrigerator for about 30 minutes (or in the freezer for 5 minutes). It should make the dough easier to handle.

6. **Peel away.** If you have cut out shapes but are finding them difficult to lift up from the parchment onto the prepared baking sheet, you can pop the rolled-out dough on a portable flat surface, such as a cutting board, and place it in the freezer for 5 minutes. Or, rather than trying to peel the shapes off the parchment, peel the surrounding dough away from the shapes and then peel the paper away from under each cut-out shape. It will keep the cut-out shape from stretching or breaking during the transfer.

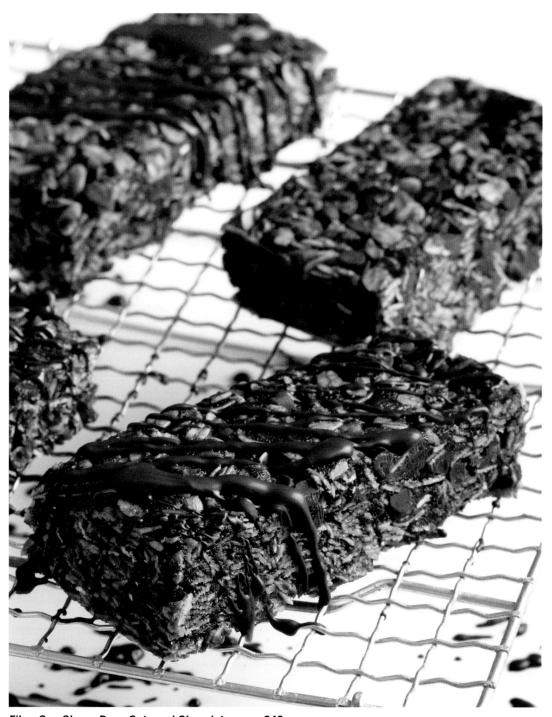

Fiber One Chewy Bars, Oats and Chocolate, page 249

Shoestring Savings

The blog that I began way back in 2009 (a hundred years ago in Internet time!) is called *Gluten-Free on a Shoestring*. You can still find me there most days of the week, at http://glutenfreeonashoestring.com/. From the beginning, I've provided reliable recipes for really good gluten-free food that anyone can make at home, inexpensively. If there are favorite comfort foods you miss now that you're eating (or just cooking and baking) gluten-free, I want to help you make them again. Nothing too fancy! But "inexpensive" has always been a relative term.

Gluten-free baking is always going to be somewhat more expensive than conventional, gluten-containing baking, because the most basic ingredients cost more. However, baking at home with the right recipes and ingredients will save you plenty. Packaged (or even bakery-made) gluten-free baked goods are typically *much* more expensive than their conventional analogs (if they are even available anywhere at all for purchase) and tend to be of inferior quality. This fact is perhaps most apparent in these recipes for "nostalgic" snacks that simply aren't available (and likely won't ever be made available) gluten-free. As much as the gluten-free market has grown, it's still a niche with a relatively large barrier to entry (dedicated gluten-free facilities! new FDA regulations!). This is all to say that, if we want moist and tender, well-priced gluten-free Hostess-style chocolate cupcakes (see page 131), we're going to have to make them ourselves! But they'll be less expensive and better than you ever imagined.

Making the recipe yourself can mean saving up to 77 percent of the cost. For example, Little Debbie Oatmeal Creme Pies (page 115) are 69¢ each to make, whereas a ready-made gluten-free version would cost $3.00 each. Make those Hostess-style cupcakes on page 131 and you'll spend 90¢ per cupcake. To buy a ready-made gluten-free version would set you back a full $3.50 per cupcake, so you'll save 74 percent by making them yourself. Strawberry Pop-Tarts (page 223) cost 39¢ each to make. Ready-made? Try $1.10 each (a cost savings of 65 percent). Brownie Bites (page 127) cost only 12¢ each to make, versus 60¢ each to buy (80 percent cost savings). Graham Crackers (page 195) cost 18¢ each to make, and 34¢ each to buy (a more modest 47 percent savings). And, of course, the taste, texture, and quality of what you make at home will be head and shoulders above the purchased products, if you can even find them for purchase.

Because this is a gluten-free baking book, these recipes call for flours of one sort or another. As part of an ongoing effort to make gluten-free baking accessible, I have always baked primarily with all-purpose gluten-free flour blends (see pages 2–8 for a full discussion of gluten-free flours and blends). Such blends are traditionally rice based, as rice flour blends are best able to mimic the behavior of conventional all-purpose wheat flours, resulting in baked goods that are indistinguishable from their conventional counterparts.

If a baked good tastes "gluten-free," as compared to just simply delicious, it's just not good enough. Gone are the days when a gluten-free muffin that falls apart in your hands was the best we could do. That gluten-free taste and texture is typically due to the fact that a baked good is dry and crumbly (the result of a poor, unbalanced recipe) or gritty (the result of gritty rice flour). That's why you need rigorously tested recipes that work (like mine!) and a flour blend based upon superfine rice flour (see page 7). Certified gluten-free superfine rice flours are, however, expensive when purchased separately (see page 5). To keep down the cost of your all-purpose gluten-free flour blend, my best advice is actually to purchase what I consider to be the most versatile gluten-free flour blend available, and buy it in bulk: Better Batter Gluten Free All Purpose Flour (see page 3). Not only does Better Batter use superfine rice flour, but as of the printing of this book, purchasing this all-purpose flour blend in bulk costs about $1.00 per 140-gram cup (including flat-rate shipping of $8.00 within the United States). My Mock Better Batter Gluten Free All Purpose Flour Blend (see page 7) costs about $1.80 per 140-gram cup. To build the few other gluten-free flours necessary to make the remaining recipes in this book (see pages 7–8), or if you do decide to build your own all-purpose blend, aim to buy the component flours in bulk whenever possible (see Resources, pages 294–296).

One more note about baking gluten-free: Whether you make your own basic all-purpose blend or buy it ready-made, try to keep it assembled and within reach in your kitchen. That way, when you're paging through these photos and recipes and inspiration strikes, you can get baking!

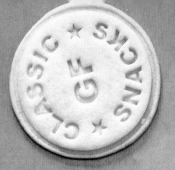
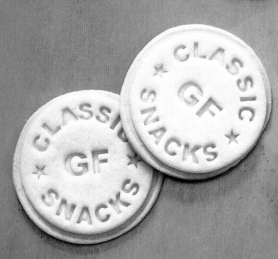
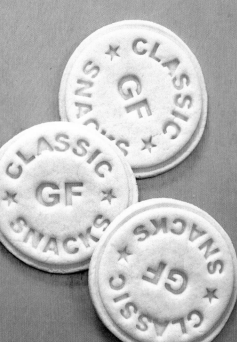
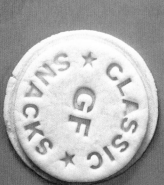
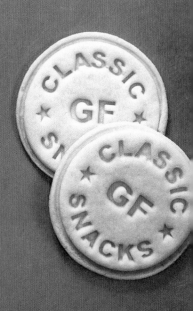
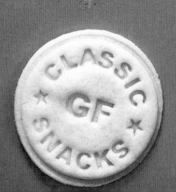

CHAPTER 2

Cookies

The Girl Scouts Have Nothing on Us (Now)!

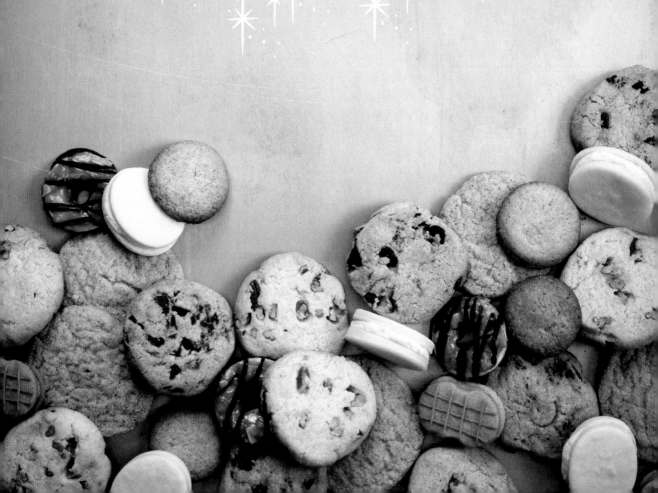

Savannah Smiles Girl Scout Cookies

MAKES ABOUT 40 COOKIES

Cookies

1¾ cups (245 g) all-purpose gluten-free flour (see page 2)

¼ cup (36 g) cornstarch

½ teaspoon baking powder

¼ teaspoon kosher salt

1 cup (115 g) confectioners' sugar

8 tablespoons (112 g) unsalted butter, at room temperature

2 teaspoons pure lemon extract

2 tablespoons water, plus more by half-teaspoonful until the dough comes together

Topping

Freshly squeezed lemon juice, for brushing

1 cup (115 g) confectioners' sugar

*B*ecause not every Girl Scout Cookie is available in every US market, I shall take this opportunity to clear up any confusion about the little cookies that set the snack world on fire once a year. Savannah Smiles are half-moon-shaped crispy lemon cookies. They're not crunchy like a cracker. They're crisp like an Oreo (page 53). There's plenty of lemon flavor in the cookies, and after they're baked, they're brushed with lemon juice and dusted in confectioners' sugar. I'm not 100 percent sure if they're called "Smiles" because they make you smile or because each cookie looks a bit like a smile. But both are equally true.

Prepare the cookies: Preheat your oven to 325°F. Line rimmed baking sheets with unbleached parchment paper and set them aside.

In a large bowl, place the flour, cornstarch, baking powder, salt, and confectioners' sugar, and whisk to combine well. Create a well in the center of the dry ingredients and add the butter, lemon extract, and 2 tablespoons of water, mixing to combine after each addition. Knead the dough with your hands, adding water by the half-teaspoonful as necessary to bring the dough together.

Transfer the dough to a large piece of unbleached parchment paper and shape it into a cylinder that is about 2 inches in diameter. Roll the cylinder tightly in the parchment paper and cinch the ends to seal it. Allow the dough to sit for 10 minutes at room temperature.

Unwrap the dough and slice it by cross-section into disks each about ¼ inch thick. Slice each round in half into a half-moon, and place about 1 inch apart from one another on the prepared baking sheets.

Place the baking sheets, one at a time, in the center of the preheated oven and bake until the cookies are just beginning to brown around the edges and are dry to the touch, about 11 minutes. Remove from the oven and allow to cool on the baking sheets for 5 minutes.

Add the topping: While still warm from the oven, brush the tops of the cookies with the lemon juice, then toss lightly in a bowl of the confectioners' sugar until well coated.

The cookies can be stored in a sealed glass container at room temperature and should maintain their texture for at least 5 days. For longer storage, seal them tightly in a freezer-safe wrap or bag, and freeze for up to 2 months. Defrost at room temperature.

Samoas Girl Scout Cookies (a.k.a. Caramel deLites)

Cookies

1¾ cups (245 g) all-purpose gluten-free flour (see page 2)

⅛ teaspoon kosher salt

½ cup (100 g) granulated sugar

8 tablespoons (112 g) unsalted butter, at room temperature

1 to 2 tablespoons (½ to 1 fluid ounce) lukewarm water

Coconut Caramel

2 cups (160 g) unsweetened coconut flakes

8 ounces Soft Caramel for Candies (page 291)

1 to 3 tablespoons milk, as necessary

Chocolate Glaze

8 ounces semisweet chocolate, chopped

2 tablespoons (28 g) virgin coconut oil

*Y*ou know how some people swear that they just don't like coconut? Well, I'm convinced that it's because they have only had the shredded, sweetened grocery store kind of coconut. The kind that makes you feel as if you're flossing your teeth with sugar. When a recipe requires dried coconut, I always reach for coconut flakes. Also sometimes referred to as coconut chips, coconut flakes are the wide, flat, dried coconut pieces that have a wonderful untoasted texture. Give the coconut flakes a quick spin on a baking tray in a low-heat oven and not only will your Samoas-style cookies taste warm, nutty, and even better than the original, your whole house will smell like heaven.

Prepare the cookies: Preheat your oven to 325°F. Line a rimmed baking sheet with unbleached parchment paper and set it aside.

In a large bowl, place the flour, salt, and sugar, and whisk to combine well. Add the butter and 1 tablespoon of the water, and mix to combine. Knead the dough together with your hands, adding more water by the quarter-teaspoonful as necessary to bring the dough together.

Place the dough between two sheets of unbleached parchment paper and roll it out until it is a bit more than ⅛ inch thick. Cut out rounds of dough with a 2-inch cookie cutter, then cut out a ½-inch circle in the center with either a ½-inch cookie cutter or the underside of a pastry tip. Gather and reroll the scraps to cut out more cookies until you've used up the dough. Transfer the cookie cutouts carefully to the prepared baking sheet. If the cutouts are fragile and too difficult to handle, place them in the refrigerator until firm before moving.

Place the baking sheet in the center of the preheated oven and bake until the cookies are set and just beginning to brown around the edges, about 8 minutes. Allow to cool for 5 minutes on the baking sheet until they are firm enough to transfer to a wire rack to cool completely. Reduce the oven temperature to 275°F.

While the cookies are cooling, prepare the coconut caramel: First, toast the coconut. Arrange the coconut flakes in a single layer on a rimmed baking sheet, place in the center of the 275°F oven, and bake until the flakes are lightly golden brown, stirring at least once (about 7 minutes). Remove the flakes from the oven and allow to cool slightly before crushing the toasted flakes in your hands. Set aside. Next, place the caramel and 1 tablespoon of milk in a medium-size, heat-safe bowl and melt them in your microwave on 70% power at 30-second intervals, stirring between intervals, until melted and smooth (or in a small, heavy-bottomed saucepan over medium-low heat). Add more milk to the melted caramels as necessary to thin the liquid to a thickly pourable consistency.

Dip one side of each cooled cookie lightly in the melted caramel mixture, and place, caramel-dipped side up, on a piece of parchment paper. Add the toasted and crushed coconut chips to the rest of the melted caramel mixture and mix to combine. With a butter knife or small offset spatula, spread the coconut mixture on top of the caramel layer on each cookie in a single layer a bit more than $1/8$ inch thick. Allow the cookie to sit at room temperature until the caramel is set, about 10 minutes.

While the caramel sets, prepare the glaze: In a medium-size, heat-safe bowl, place the chocolate and coconut oil and melt according to the instructions on page 21. Allow the chocolate to sit at room temperature until it begins to thicken a bit. Carefully dip the bottom of each cookie in the melted chocolate, and place the cookie, chocolate side down, back on the parchment paper. Drizzle a bit more chocolate over the top of each cookie in a zigzag pattern. Allow to sit at room temperature until the chocolate is set.

These cookies are best enjoyed the day they are assembled or for a couple days after. For longer storage, seal the plain shortbread cookies tightly in a freezer-safe wrap or bag, and freeze for up to 2 months. Defrost at room temperature, and then finish with the coconut, caramel, and glaze as directed.

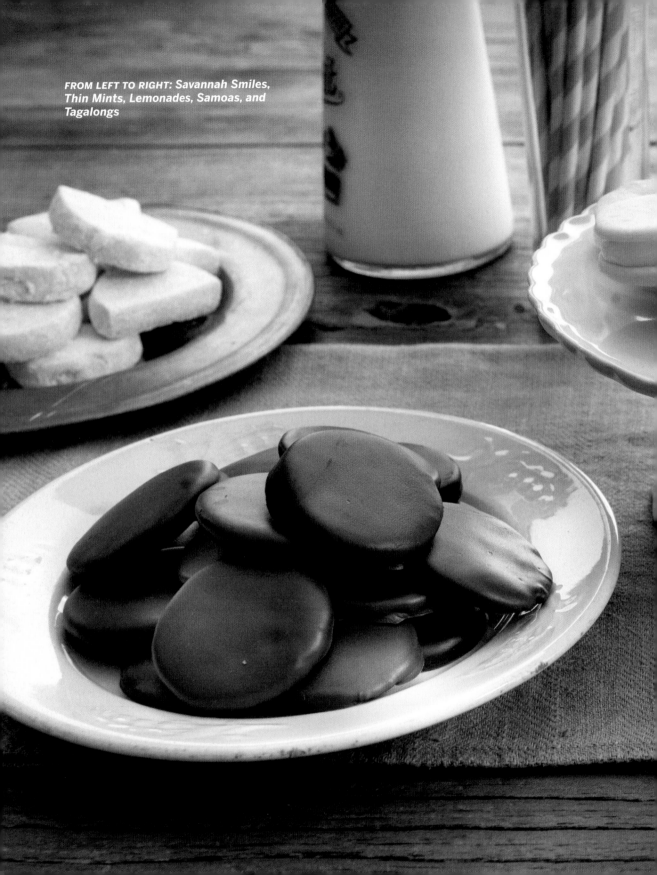

*FROM LEFT TO RIGHT: Savannah Smiles,
Thin Mints, Lemonades, Samoas, and
Tagalongs*

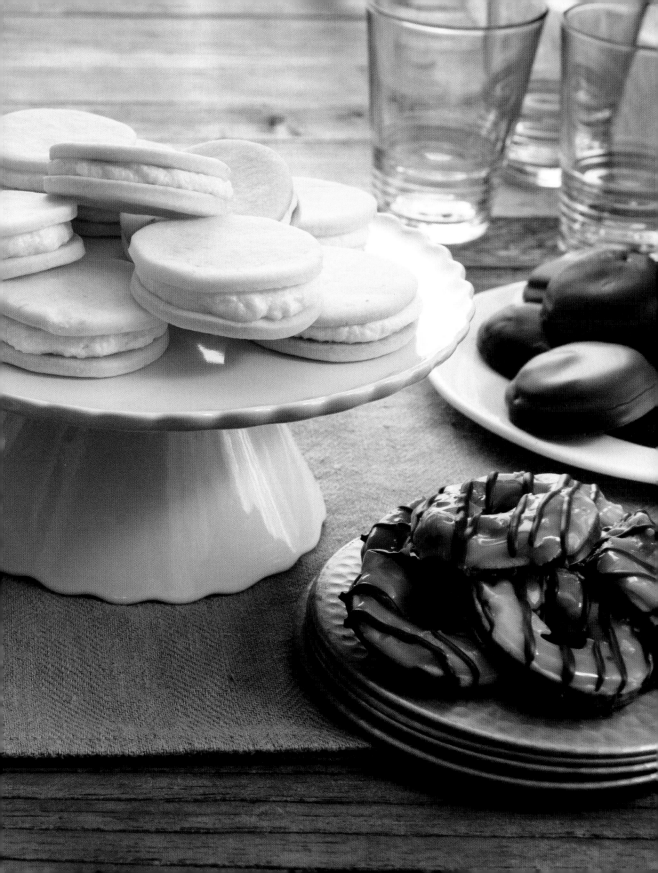

Tagalongs Girl Scout Cookies (a.k.a. Peanut Butter Patties)

MAKES 24 COOKIES

Cookies

1¾ cups (245 g) all-purpose gluten-free flour (see page 2)

⅛ teaspoon kosher salt

½ cup (100 g) granulated sugar

8 tablespoons (112 g) unsalted butter, at room temperature

1 teaspoon pure vanilla extract

1 to 2 tablespoons (½ to 1 fluid ounce) lukewarm water

Filling

Peanut Butter Filling (page 110)

Chocolate Glaze

14 ounces semisweet chocolate, chopped

3 tablespoons (42 g) virgin coconut oil

Although I'm really not sure why these are called Tagalongs, the plain, descriptive name "Peanut Butter Patties" doesn't really convey how special these deceptively simple shortbread cookies with peanut butter crème are. The crisp but tender shortbread, topped with a smooth peanut butter filling, covered in a rich chocolate glaze is like a cookie version of a Reese's Peanut Butter Cup.

Prepare the cookies: Preheat your oven to 325°F. Line a rimmed baking sheet with unbleached parchment paper and set it aside.

In a large bowl, place the flour, salt, and sugar, and whisk to combine well. Add the butter, vanilla, and 1 tablespoon of the water, and mix to combine. Knead the dough together with your hands, adding more water by the quarter-teaspoonful as necessary to bring the dough together. Place the dough between two sheets of unbleached parchment paper and roll it out until it is a bit more than ⅛ inch thick. Cut out rounds of dough with a 2-inch cookie cutter. Gather and reroll the scraps to cut out more cookies until you've used up the dough. Transfer the cookie cutouts carefully to the prepared baking sheet. If they are fragile and too difficult to handle, place the cutouts in the refrigerator until firm before moving them.

Place the baking sheet in the center of the preheated oven and bake until the cookies are set and just beginning to brown around the edges, about 8 minutes. As soon as the cookies come out of the oven, press down gently on the top of each cookie with your thumb or a small spoon to create a shallow impression about 1½ inches in diameter in the center of the cookie. This will create a well for the filling. Allow the cookies to cool for 5 minutes on the baking sheet, until they are firm enough to transfer to a wire rack to cool completely.

Prepare the Peanut Butter Filling. Place the cooled cookies on a baking sheet in a single layer. Place the filling in a pastry bag fitted with a ¼-inch plain pastry tip. Pipe a generous amount of filling in a single, even layer on top of each cooled cookie into the slight impression you made previously. With wet fingers, press down the filling if necessary. Allow the filling to set at room temperature until stable, about 30 minutes.

Once the cookies are cool, prepare the glaze: In a medium-size, microwave-safe bowl, place the chocolate and coconut oil and melt according to the instructions on page 21. Allow the chocolate to sit at room temperature until it begins to thicken a bit. Immerse the cookies, one at a time, in the glaze. Press down on the cookie with the tines of a fork, then flip it gently in the chocolate. Pull the cookie out of the chocolate by slipping the fork under it and bobbing the cookie on the surface of the chocolate a few times before pulling it along the edge of the bowl and carefully placing it on a clean sheet of waxed or parchment paper. Allow the glaze to set at room temperature.

These cookies are best enjoyed the day they have been dipped in the chocolate glaze. The finished cookies can be stored in a sealed glass container at room temperature for about 2 days. For longer storage, seal the finished cookies tightly in a freezer-safe wrap or bag, and freeze for up to 2 months. Defrost at room temperature. The chocolate coating may bloom a bit over time, but it won't affect the taste at all.

Thin Mints Girl Scout Cookies

MAKES ABOUT 70 COOKIES

Cookies

5 tablespoons (70 g) unsalted butter

4 ounces semisweet chocolate, chopped

¼ teaspoon pure vanilla extract

½ teaspoon pure peppermint extract

¾ cup (105 g) all-purpose gluten-free flour (see page 2)

½ cup (40 g) unsweetened cocoa powder

¼ teaspoon baking soda

½ teaspoon kosher salt

½ cup (100 g) granulated sugar

Warm water by the quarter-teaspoonful, as necessary

While I was growing up, Thin Mints were always my favorite Girl Scout Cookie, and somehow it mattered to me that my tastes were so unoriginal and uninspired. Everybody loves Thin Mints! Now I'm a grown, married woman with three children, and I am finally confident enough to own my ordinary choices. Snappy, minty, chocolaty goodness, these Thin Mint–style cookies taste like everything you remember about Thin Mints, but they're safely gluten-free. One might even say they're extraordinary in how ordinary they actually are.

Prepare the cookies: Preheat your oven to 300°F. Line rimmed baking sheets with unbleached parchment paper and set them aside.

In a medium-size, microwave-safe bowl, place the butter and chocolate and melt according to the instructions on page 21. Stir in the vanilla and peppermint extracts, and set the bowl aside. In a large bowl, place the flour, cocoa powder, baking soda, salt, and sugar, and whisk to combine well. Create a well in the center of the dry ingredients, add the melted chocolate mixture, and mix to combine. Knead the dough together, adding water by the quarter-teaspoonful as necessary to bring the dough together and make sure that it is pliable and not stiff.

Place the dough between two sheets of unbleached parchment paper, and roll it out until it is about ¼ inch thick. Cut out rounds that are about 1¾ inches in diameter, and place them about 1 inch apart from one another on the prepared baking sheets. Gather and reroll the scraps to cut out more cookies until you've used up the dough. Chill until firm to help the cookies bake more evenly.

Place the baking sheets in the center of the preheated oven and bake for 7 minutes, or until the cookies are dry to the touch. Remove from the oven, and allow the cookies to cool completely on the baking sheets.

Once the cookies are cool, prepare the glaze: In a medium-size, heat-safe bowl, place the dark chocolate and coconut oil and melt according to the instructions on page 21. Add the peppermint extract, and mix to incorporate. Allow the chocolate to sit at room temperature until it begins to thicken a bit. Line a rimmed baking sheet with unbleached parchment or waxed paper, and set it just to the side. Immerse the cookies, one at a time, in the glaze. Press down on the cookie with the tines of a fork, then flip it gently in the chocolate. Pull the cookie out of the chocolate by slipping the fork under it and bobbing the cookie on the surface of the chocolate a few times before pulling it along the edge of the bowl and carefully placing it on the prepared baking sheet. Allow the chocolate glaze to set at room temperature.

These cookies are best enjoyed the day they have been dipped in the chocolate glaze. The finished cookies can be stored in a sealed glass container at room temperature for about 2 days. For longer storage, seal the finished cookies tightly in a freezer-safe wrap or bag, and freeze for up to 2 months. Defrost at room temperature. The chocolate coating may bloom a bit over time, but it won't affect the taste at all.

Chocolate Peppermint Glaze

14 ounces dark chocolate, chopped

3 tablespoons (42 g) virgin coconut oil

¼ to ½ teaspoon pure peppermint extract, to taste

Lemonades Girl Scout Cookies

MAKES ABOUT 20 SANDWICH COOKIES

Cookies

1½ cups (210 g) gluten-free cake flour (see page 2)

½ cup (58 g) confectioners' sugar

¼ teaspoon kosher salt

Zest and juice of 1 lemon (about 3 tablespoons juice)

8 tablespoons (112 g) unsalted butter, at room temperature

1 egg (50 g, weighed out of the shell), at room temperature, beaten

Water by the quarter-teaspoonful, as necessary

Filling

Stiff Sandwich Cookie Filling, Lemon Variation (page 109)

Another brilliant lemon Girl Scout creation, Lemonades are lemon sandwich cookies with a lemon filling. They have the tender texture of a Vienna Finger (page 93), but both the cookies and the filling are properly lemony: not enough to make you pucker but enough that the cookies are bright and fresh-tasting.

Prepare the cookies: Preheat your oven to 325°F. Line rimmed baking sheets with unbleached parchment paper and set them aside.

In a large bowl, place the flour, confectioners' sugar, salt, and lemon zest, and whisk to combine well, breaking up any clumps in the lemon zest, which tends to stick to itself. Add the lemon juice, butter, and then the egg, mixing to combine after each addition. The dough will come together and should be smooth and relatively thick. Knead the dough if necessary, adding water by the quarter-teaspoonful as needed to bring the dough together. Place the dough between two sheets of unbleached parchment paper and roll into a rectangle a bit more than ⅛ inch thick. Set on a flat surface and place in the freezer until firm, about 5 minutes.

Once the cookie dough is chilled, cut out rounds using a 2¼-inch round cookie cutter. Place the cutouts less than an inch apart from one another on the prepared baking sheets (they will not spread during baking). Gather and reroll the scraps to cut out more cookies until you've used up the dough. Place the baking sheets, one at a time, in the center of the preheated oven and bake until the cookies are just beginning to brown around the edges, about 10 minutes. Remove from the oven and allow the cookies to cool on the baking sheet for 5 minutes, then transfer to a wire rack to cool completely.

Prepare the Lemon Stiff Sandwich Cookie Filling. Transfer the filling to a pastry bag fitted with a ¼-inch plain piping tip. Once the cookies are cool, invert half of the cookies, and pipe a generous amount of filling in a single layer on each inverted cookie. Top with the remaining cookies and press down gently to form a sandwich. Allow to sit until the filling is set.

The filled cookies can be stored in a sealed glass container at room temperature and should maintain their texture for at least 5 days. For longer storage, seal the unfilled lemon wafers tightly in a freezer-safe wrap or bag, and freeze for up to 2 months. Defrost at room temperature and fill as directed.

Do-Si-Dos Girl Scout Cookies (a.k.a. Peanut Butter Sandwiches)

MAKES 15 SANDWICH COOKIES

Cookies

13 tablespoons (182 g) unsalted butter

1 cup (256 g) no-stir smooth peanut butter

1½ cups (210 g) all-purpose gluten-free flour (see page 2)

1 teaspoon baking powder

½ teaspoon baking soda

½ teaspoon kosher salt

½ cup (100 g) granulated sugar

½ cup (109 g) packed light brown sugar

¾ cup (75 g) certified gluten-free old-fashioned rolled oats

1½ teaspoons pure vanilla extract

1 egg (50 g, weighed out of shell), at room temperature, beaten

*B*aking cookies with peanut butter in the cookie batter tends to make for crunchy cookies. Baking with oats tends to make for soft cookies. Put the two together in these cookies and you have the perfect balance of tender and crunchy. The peanut butter filling in the center helps make these cookie sandwiches an event worth savoring. You can poke a hole in the center of the top cookies when they come out of the oven so they look just like the real thing, but that is strictly optional.

Prepare the cookies: Preheat your oven to 325°F. Line rimmed baking sheets with parchment paper and set them aside.

In a small, heavy-bottomed saucepan, heat the butter and peanut butter over medium heat, stirring frequently, until just melted. Remove the pan from the heat, and set it aside to cool briefly. In a large bowl, place the flour, baking powder, baking soda, salt, and granulated sugar, and whisk to combine well. Add the brown sugar, and whisk again, working out any lumps. Add the oats, and stir to combine. Create a well in the center of the dry ingredients, add the melted peanut butter mixture, and mix to combine. Add the vanilla and the egg, and mix once again to combine. The dough will be thick but soft. With wet hands, divide the dough into about 30 pieces, each about 1 tablespoon. Roll each into a ball, and press flat between wet palms. Place the disks on the prepared baking sheets about 2 inches apart (they will spread during baking). Place the baking sheets with the cookie dough on them in the freezer until firm, about 10 minutes.

Once the dough is chilled, place the baking sheets, one at a time, in the center of the preheated oven and bake until the cookies are lightly golden brown all over and a bit darker around the edges, about 10 minutes. Remove from the oven and, if desired, poke a small hole through the center of half of the cookies with a toothpick. Allow to cool on the baking sheet until set, about 10 minutes, before transferring to a wire rack to cool completely.

Prepare the Peanut Butter Filling. Transfer the filling to a pastry bag fitted with a ¼-inch plain pastry tip. Once the cookies are completely cool, invert half of the cooled cookies (the half without holes, if you made holes), and pipe a generous amount of filling on each inverted cookie. Top with the rest of the cookies and press gently to form a sandwich. Allow to sit at room temperature (or in the refrigerator) until the filling is set.

The filled cookies can be stored in a sealed glass container at room temperature and should maintain their texture for at least 5 days. For longer storage, seal the filled sandwich cookies tightly in a freezer-safe wrap or bag, and freeze for up to 2 months. Defrost at room temperature.

Filling

**Peanut Butter Filling
(page 110)**

———————

Thanks-A-Lot Girl Scout Cookies

MAKES ABOUT 50 COOKIES

Cookies

1¾ cups (245 g) all-purpose gluten-free flour (see page 2)

5 tablespoons (45 g) cornstarch

⅛ teaspoon baking soda

¼ teaspoon kosher salt

1 cup (115 g) confectioners' sugar

8 tablespoons (112 g) unsalted butter, at room temperature

1 egg white (25 g), at room temperature

2 tablespoons (1 fluid ounce) warm milk or water

Chocolate Glaze

8 ounces semisweet chocolate, chopped

2 tablespoons (28 g) virgin coconut oil

*T*hanks-A-Lot cookies are crisp, buttery shortbread cookies dipped in rich chocolate. Everybody knows that Girl Scout Thanks-A-Lots have "Thank You" embossed on the cookie. If you'd like to shoot for total authenticity, there are all kinds of cookie stamps available from various sellers on Etsy. com, including some that will make custom stamps with whatever image or saying you like. But, according to the Girl Scouts, they also make them with this most gracious, simple sentiment in Spanish, French, Chinese, and Swahili. How perfectly cosmopolitan of them.

Prepare the cookies: Preheat your oven to 325°F. Line rimmed baking sheets with unbleached parchment paper and set them aside.

In a large bowl, place the flour, cornstarch, baking soda, salt, and confectioners' sugar, and whisk to combine well. Create a well in the center of the dry ingredients and add the butter, egg white, and milk, mixing to combine after each addition. The dough will come together and should be smooth, but soft. Wrap the dough in plastic wrap and place it in the refrigerator for 10 minutes or allow it to sit at room temperature for about 30 minutes, or until it has begun to firm up.

Unwrap the dough, place it on a flat surface, and roll it into a rectangle that is a bit more than ⅛ inch thick. If the dough seems too sticky to handle, return it to the refrigerator to chill until more firm (but not too firm to roll out). Cut out rounds with a cookie cutter that is about 2½ inches in diameter. Place the rounds about 1 inch apart on the prepared baking sheets (they will not spread during baking). Gather and reroll the scraps to cut out more cookies until you've used up the dough.

Place the baking sheets, one at a time, in the center of the preheated oven and bake until the cookies are just beginning to brown around the edges, about 9 minutes. Remove from the oven and allow to cool on the baking sheet for 5 minutes before transferring to a wire rack to cool completely.

Once the cookies are cool, prepare the glaze: Line a rimmed baking sheet with parchment or waxed paper, and set it aside. In a medium-size, heat-safe bowl, place the chocolate and coconut oil and melt according to the instructions on page 21. Allow the chocolate to sit at room temperature until it begins to thicken a bit. To decorate the cookies, spoon some of the melted chocolate mixture onto the underside of each cookie, spread out the chocolate glaze to the edges, and place, chocolate side down, on the prepared baking sheet. Allow to set at room temperature, or in the refrigerator, until firm.

These cookies are best enjoyed the day they are finished with the chocolate glaze. The finished cookies can be stored in a sealed glass container at room temperature for about 2 days. For longer storage, seal the finished cookies tightly in a freezer-safe wrap or bag, and freeze for up to 2 months. Defrost at room temperature. The chocolate coating may bloom a bit over time, but it won't affect the taste at all.

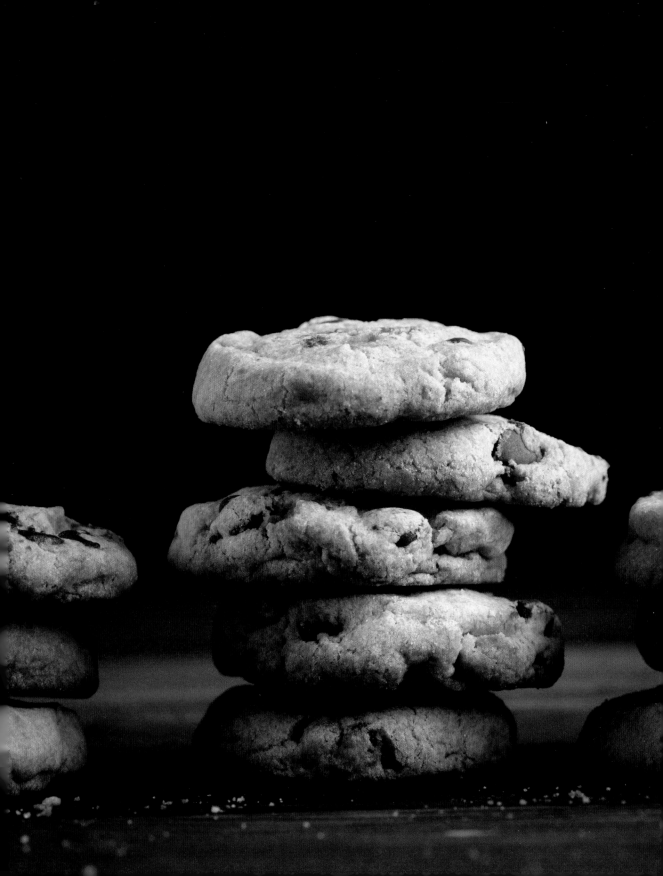

Nabisco Chips Ahoy! Cookies, Original

MAKES 16 COOKIES

*I*f you're asking yourself how *these* chocolate chip cookies taste and smell (and look!) just like the crunchy, crumbly Chips Ahoy! cookies we all know and love, and are so different from any other chocolate chip cookie, it's all about the balance of ingredients—especially the relative dryness of the dough. You can swap out butter for more shortening, and swap out the sugars, but they just won't taste and smell and look like Chips Ahoy! Chalk it up to the magic of baking. To achieve that signature thick, round shape of the original, these are slice-and-bake, not drop cookies.

Preheat your oven to 325°F. Line a rimmed baking sheet with unbleached parchment paper and set it aside.

In a large bowl, place the flour, baking soda, salt, and granulated sugar, and whisk to combine well. Add the brown sugar and whisk again, working out any lumps. Create a well in the center of the dry ingredients and add the butter and shortening, then the vanilla and egg, mixing to combine after each addition. Knead the dough together with your hands, adding water by the half-teaspoonful as necessary to bring the dough together. It will be thick. Add the cornstarch-dusted chips to the cookie dough and mix until the chips are evenly distributed throughout.

Place the dough on a large piece of unbleached parchment paper and roll in the paper into a cylinder about 2½ inches in diameter, and roll to wrap tightly, twisting the ends to seal. Place the dough in the freezer until just firm, about 10 minutes.

Remove the cookie dough from the freezer. If the cylinder of dough has lost its round shape, rock it back and forth on the counter as if it were a rolling pin to restore the round shape. Unwrap the dough and slice it with a very sharp chef's knife thickly in cross-section into rounds that are nearly ¾ inch thick. Place the rounds about 1 inch apart on the prepared baking sheet, and bake until the cookies are lightly golden

2 cups (280 g) all-purpose gluten-free flour (see page 2)

½ teaspoon baking soda

¼ teaspoon kosher salt

10 tablespoons (125 g) granulated sugar

¼ cup (55 g) packed light brown sugar

4 tablespoons (56 g) unsalted butter, at room temperature

4 tablespoons (48 g) nonhydrogenated vegetable shortening, melted and cooled

1½ teaspoons pure vanilla extract

1 egg (50 g, weighed out of shell), at room temperature, beaten

Lukewarm water by the half-teaspoonful, as necessary

9 ounces semisweet chocolate chips, tossed with 1 teaspoon cornstarch

brown all over and set in the center, about 12 minutes. Remove from the oven and allow to cool on the baking sheet for at least 10 minutes, or until stable, before transferring to a wire rack to cool completely. The cookies will crisp as they cool.

The cookies can be stored in a sealed glass container at room temperature and should maintain their texture for at least 5 days. For longer storage, seal them tightly in a freezer-safe wrap or bag, and freeze for up to 2 months. Defrost at room temperature.

Nabisco Oreo Sandwich Cookies, Chocolate

MAKES ABOUT 30 SANDWICH COOKIES

Cookies

8 tablespoons (112 g) unsalted butter, chopped

2 ounces bittersweet chocolate, chopped

1¼ cups (250 g) granulated sugar

1 egg (50 g, weighed out of shell) plus 1 egg white (25 g), at room temperature, beaten

1 teaspoon pure vanilla extract

2¼ cups (315 g) all-purpose gluten-free flour (see page 2)

1 cup (80 g) unsweetened cocoa powder

1 teaspoon baking soda

½ teaspoon baking powder

½ teaspoon kosher salt

Filling

Stiff Sandwich Cookie Filling (page 109)

*W*hy do you need to make your own Oreo-style cookies, when there are gluten-free Oreo clones already on the market? Well, the chocolate sandwich cookies on the market taste "pretty good." But they're also really expensive, and "pretty good" just isn't good enough. These sandwich cookies are made to be dunked in milk, crushed and layered in an ice-cream cake, or made into a Cookies'n'Creme Candy Bar (page 272). And they left "pretty good" behind a long time ago. For the cocoa powder in this recipe, I highly recommend using Hershey's Special Dark, as it is the darkest-colored unsweetened cocoa powder that is readily available and it makes the most authentic-looking and -tasting Oreo-style cookies.

Prepare the cookies: Preheat your oven to 325°F. Line rimmed baking sheets with unbleached parchment paper and set them aside.

In a medium-size, heat-safe bowl, place the butter and chocolate and melt as described on page 21. Add the granulated sugar to the chocolate mixture, and mix to combine. Add the egg, egg white, and vanilla, and mix to combine. Set the bowl aside.

In a large bowl, place the flour, cocoa powder, baking soda, baking powder, and salt, and whisk to combine well. Create a well in the center of the dry ingredients and add the wet mixture. Mix to combine, and then knead the dough with your hands to bring it together. Roll out the dough between two pieces of parchment paper until it is about ¼ inch thick. Place the dough, still between the sheets of parchment, on a baking sheet or cutting board, and then place it in the freezer to chill until nearly firm, about 5 minutes. Remove from the freezer, and remove the top sheet of paper. Cut out rounds with a 2-inch cookie cutter, and place them 1 inch apart from one another on the prepared baking sheets.

Place the baking sheets, one at a time, in the center of the preheated oven and bake until the cookies are dry to the touch, about 15 minutes.

Remove from the oven and allow to cool on the baking sheets. The cookies will crisp as they cool.

Prepare the Stiff Sandwich Cookie Filling. Transfer the filling to a pastry bag fitted with a ½-inch open piping tip. When the cookies are cool, invert half of the cookies and pipe about 1½ tablespoons of filling onto the inverted chocolate wafer cookies. Top with the other cookies and push down gently to form a sandwich.

The filled cookies can be stored in a sealed glass container at room temperature and should maintain their texture for at least 5 days. For longer storage, seal the unfilled chocolate wafers tightly in a freezer-safe wrap or bag, and freeze for up to 2 months. Defrost at room temperature and fill as directed.

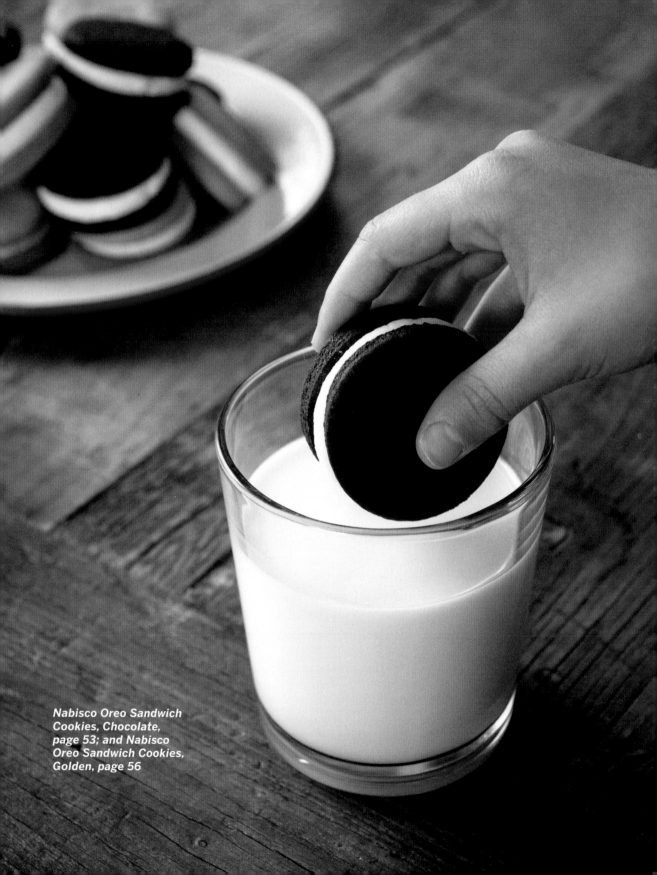

Nabisco Oreo Sandwich Cookies, Chocolate, page 53; and Nabisco Oreo Sandwich Cookies, Golden, page 56

Nabisco Oreo Sandwich Cookies, Golden

MAKES ABOUT 30 SANDWICH COOKIES

Cookies

2⅓ cups (327 g) all-purpose gluten-free flour (see page 2)

9 tablespoons (81 g) cornstarch

1 teaspoon baking soda

½ teaspoon baking powder

½ teaspoon kosher salt

1¼ cups (250 g) granulated sugar

8 tablespoons (112 g) unsalted butter, chopped

2 tablespoons (24 g) nonhydrogenated vegetable shortening

2 eggs (100 g, weighed out of shell), at room temperature, beaten

1½ teaspoons pure vanilla extract

Filling

Stiff Sandwich Cookie Filling (page 109)

*W*e *assume* that everybody loves chocolate. We even call vanilla "plain." Is that really fair, though? Golden Oreos were always a personal favorite of mine, but I was ashamed of that fact in my youth. Imagine that! If you or a member of your family is a lover of Golden Oreos, make them these vanilla beauties and celebrate them for going against the grain, being who they are, spreading their wings. After all, the recipe may be similar to that for Oreo Chocolate Sandwich Cookies (page 53), but in these the vanilla flavor really shines through.

Prepare the cookies: Preheat your oven to 325°F. Line rimmed baking sheets with unbleached parchment paper and set them aside.

In a large bowl, place the flour, cornstarch, baking soda, baking powder, salt, and sugar, and whisk to combine well. Create a well in the center of the dry ingredients and add the butter, shortening, eggs, and vanilla, and mix to combine. Then knead the dough with your hands to bring it together. Roll out the dough between two pieces of parchment paper until it is about ¼ inch thick. Place the dough, still between the sheets of parchment, on a baking sheet or cutting board, and then place it in the freezer to chill until nearly firm, about 5 minutes. Remove from the freezer, and remove the top sheet of paper. Cut out rounds with a 2-inch cookie cutter, and place them 1 inch apart from one another on the prepared baking sheets.

Place the baking sheets, one at a time, in the center of the preheated oven and bake until the cookies are dry to the touch, about 13 minutes. Remove from the oven and allow to cool on the baking sheets. The cookies will crisp as they cool.

Prepare the Stiff Sandwich Cookie Filling. Transfer the filling to a pastry bag fitted with a ½-inch open piping tip, invert half of the cookies, and pipe about 1½ tablespoons of filling on the inverted, cooled wafer cookies. Top with the other cookies and push down gently to form a sandwich.

The filled cookies can be stored in a sealed glass container at room temperature and should maintain their texture for at least 5 days. For longer storage, seal the unfilled vanilla wafers tightly in a freezer-safe wrap or bag, and freeze for up to 2 months. Defrost at room temperature and fill as directed.

Nabisco Oreo Sandwich Cookies, Golden Chocolate Creme

MAKES ABOUT 30 SANDWICH COOKIES

Cookies

2⅓ cups (327 g) all-purpose gluten-free flour (see page 2)

9 tablespoons (81 g) cornstarch

1 teaspoon baking soda

½ teaspoon baking powder

½ teaspoon kosher salt

1¼ cups (250 g) granulated sugar

8 tablespoons (112 g) unsalted butter, chopped

2 tablespoons (24 g) nonhydrogenated vegetable shortening

2 eggs (100 g, weighed out of shell), at room temperature, beaten

1 teaspoon pure vanilla extract

Filling

Stiff Sandwich Cookie Filling, Chocolate Variation (page 109)

These hybrid, chocolate-vanilla Oreo-style cookies are the best of both worlds. The golden wafers let the vanilla shine, and the flavor of the smooth chocolate creme really lingers on your tongue—especially when you twist the cookies open and steal a few licks of the filling before taking a bite.

Prepare the cookies: Preheat your oven to 325°F. Line rimmed baking sheets with unbleached parchment paper and set them aside.

In a large bowl, place the flour, cornstarch, baking soda, baking powder, salt, and sugar, and whisk to combine well. Create a well in the center of the dry ingredients and add the butter, shortening, eggs, and vanilla, and mix to combine. Then knead the dough with your hands to bring it together. Roll out the dough between two pieces of parchment paper until it is about ¼ inch thick. Place the dough, still between the sheets of parchment, on a baking sheet or cutting board, and then place it in the freezer to chill until nearly firm, about 5 minutes. Remove from the freezer, and remove the top sheet of paper. Cut out rounds with a 2-inch cookie cutter, then place 1 inch apart on the baking sheets.

Place the baking sheets, one at a time, in the center of the preheated oven and bake until the cookies are dry to the touch, about 13 minutes. Remove from the oven and allow to cool on the baking sheets. The cookies will crisp as they cool.

Prepare the Chocolate Stiff Sandwich Cookie Filling. Transfer it to a pastry bag fitted with a ½-inch open piping tip, invert half of the cookies, and pipe about 1½ tablespoons of filling on the inverted, cooled wafer cookies. Top with the other cookies and push down gently to sandwich.

The filled cookies can be stored in a sealed glass container at room temperature and should maintain their texture for at least 5 days. For longer storage, seal the unfilled vanilla wafers tightly in a freezer-safe wrap or bag, and freeze for up to 2 months. Defrost at room temperature and fill as directed.

Nabisco Nutter Butter Peanut Butter Sandwich Cookies

MAKES 40 SANDWICH COOKIES

I'm not gonna lie: The stripes on these Nutter Butter–style peanut butter sandwich cookies are a bit labor-intensive and perhaps unnecessary. But I had to at least *show* them to you as some sort of visual proof that these cookies are, simply put, a dead ringer for the original. Tender and crisp, with that nutty-sweet filling, these are what Nutter Butters taste like. If you've never had a gluten-filled version, feed this gluten-free version to a gluten-eating friend side by side. Like the Pepsi challenge but with cookies. If you are not up for it, feel free to skip the extra step involved in making the crisscross pattern. Just use up all the cookie dough in making the cookies themselves. And a no-stir peanut butter (the kind that doesn't separate in the jar) will provide the proper results.

Prepare the cookies: Preheat your oven to 325°F. Line rimmed baking sheets with unbleached parchment paper and set them aside.

In a small, heavy-bottomed saucepan, place the peanut butter and butter over medium heat, stirring frequently until melted and smooth. Remove from the heat and set aside to cool briefly. In a large bowl, place the flour, baking powder, baking soda, salt, and granulated sugar, and whisk to combine well. Add the brown sugar, whisking to combine well and working out any lumps. Create a well in the center of the dry ingredients, add the melted peanut butter mixture, and stir to combine. Add the egg and vanilla, and mix until the dough comes together. Knead with your hands until smooth. The dough should be thick but soft.

Place the cookie dough between two sheets of unbleached parchment paper, and roll out into a rectangle about ¼ inch thick. Remove the top sheet of paper, and cut out oval shapes with a 2-inch oval cookie

Cookies

1 cup (256 g) no-stir smooth peanut butter

8 tablespoons (112 g) unsalted butter

2 cups (280 g) all-purpose gluten-free flour (see page 2)

1 teaspoon baking powder

½ teaspoon baking soda

½ teaspoon kosher salt

½ cup (100 g) granulated sugar

½ cup (109 g) packed light brown sugar

1 egg (50 g, weighed out of shell), at room temperature, beaten

1 teaspoon pure vanilla extract

Hot water by the tablespoonful, as needed

CONTINUED ON PAGE 60

CONTINUED FROM PAGE 59

Filling

**Peanut Butter Filling
(page 110)**

cutter. Place the shapes about 1 inch apart on the prepared baking sheets. Gather and reroll the scraps, reserving about ¼ cup of dough. With a moistened thumb and forefinger, carefully pinch each oval on either side of the width of each oval's center to create a peanut shape.

Place the reserved dough in a small bowl and mix with hot water by the tablespoon, stirring until you have a thick paste. Transfer the paste to a pastry bag fitted with a small open pastry tip (such as the #2 tip), and pipe a crisscross pattern on half of the cutouts. Place the baking sheets in the freezer until the cutouts are firm, about 5 minutes.

Place the baking sheets, one at a time, in the center of the preheated oven and bake until the cookies are lightly golden brown all over, about 9 minutes. Remove from the oven and allow to cool completely on the baking sheets.

Prepare the Peanut Butter Filling. Transfer the filling to a pastry bag fitted with a ¼-inch plain piping tip. Invert the half of the cookies that are without the crisscross pattern, and pipe a generous amount of filling onto each overturned cookie. Top with the decorated cookies, pressing down gently to form a sandwich. Allow to sit at room temperature (or in the refrigerator) until the filling is set.

The filled cookies can be stored in a sealed glass container at room temperature and should maintain their texture for at least 5 days. For longer storage, seal the unfilled peanut butter cookies tightly in a freezer-safe wrap or bag, and freeze for up to 2 months. Defrost at room temperature and fill as directed. If the cookies get knocked around during freezing, the crisscross pattern on half of the cookies may get disturbed.

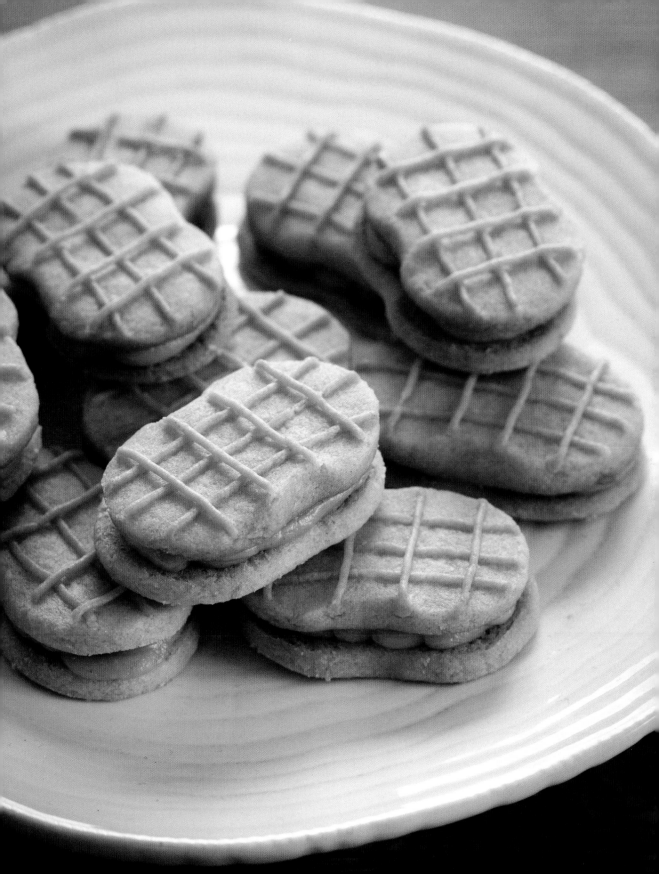

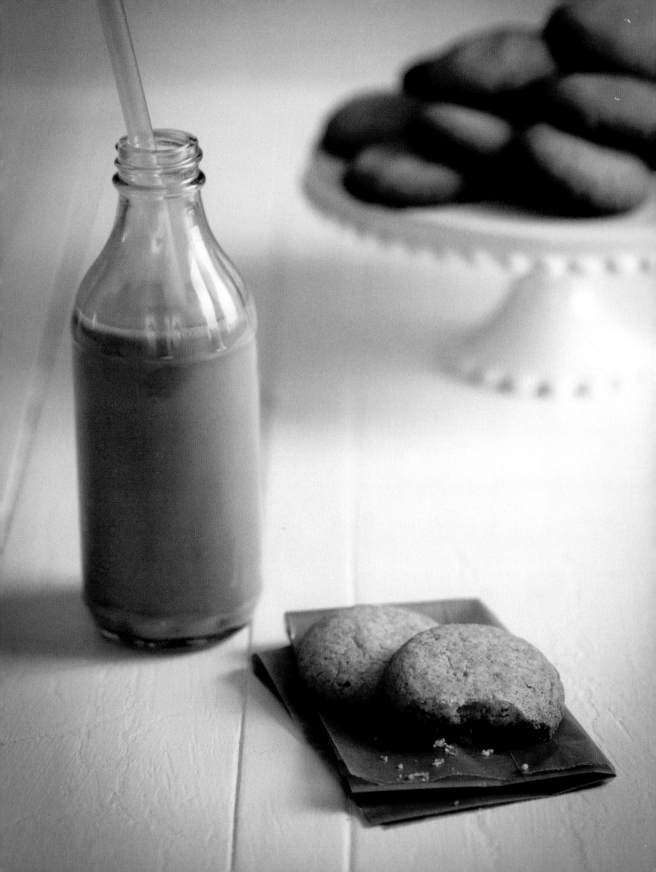

Nabisco Nilla Wafers

MAKES 24 WAFERS

*E*ven self-proclaimed chocolate lovers have no choice but to love a Nilla Wafer. Deep vanilla flavor in a crispy, crunchy little cookie so perfectly nostalgic that they wouldn't dare change the packaging. Nilla Wafers are the sort of cookie that we all take for granted—until, suddenly, we can no longer have them. Making your own is super simple, and if you can't be bothered piping the dough onto the baking sheet to get perfectly round cookies, just scoop it by the rounded tablespoonful.

Preheat your oven to 325°F. Line rimmed baking sheets with unbleached parchment paper and set them aside.

In a large bowl, place the flour, baking powder, baking soda, and salt, and whisk to combine. Add the butter, brown sugar, egg, vanilla, and milk, mixing thoroughly after each addition. The batter should still be thin enough to be piped through a plain pastry piping tip, but not runny.

Transfer the dough to a pastry bag fitted with a ¼-inch plain piping tip and pipe 1-inch rounds, spaced about 1 inch apart from one another, onto the prepared baking sheets. The cookies will spread, but not a lot. With wet fingers, gently flatten the top of each raw cookie to smooth any peaks left after piping. Chill the raw cookies on the baking sheet in the freezer for about 5 minutes until firm.

Once the raw cookies are firm, place the baking sheets, one at a time, in the center of the preheated oven and bake until the cookies are golden brown all over, 15 to 17 minutes. Allow to cool for 5 minutes on the baking sheets before transferring to a wire rack to cool completely. They will crisp as they cool.

The cookies can be stored in a sealed glass container at room temperature and should maintain their texture for at least 5 days. For longer storage, seal them tightly in a freezer-safe wrap or bag, and freeze for up to 2 months. Defrost at room temperature.

1⅓ cups (187 g) all-purpose gluten-free flour (see page 2)

½ teaspoon baking powder

⅛ teaspoon baking soda

½ teaspoon kosher salt

8 tablespoons (112 g) unsalted butter, at room temperature

½ cup (109 g) packed light brown sugar

1 egg (50 g, weighed out of shell), at room temperature, beaten

4 teaspoons pure vanilla extract

2 tablespoons (1 fluid ounce) milk

Nabisco Ginger Snaps

MAKES ABOUT 35 COOKIES

1½ cups (210 g) all-purpose gluten-free flour (see page 2)

¼ cup (36 g) cornstarch

¾ teaspoon baking soda

1½ teaspoons ground cinnamon

1 teaspoon ground ginger

¼ teaspoon kosher salt

¼ cup (50 g) granulated sugar

⅓ cup (73 g) packed light brown sugar

5 tablespoons (70 g) unsalted butter, at room temperature

3 tablespoons (63 g) unsulfured molasses

2 tablespoons (42 g) honey

½ teaspoon pure vanilla extract

1 egg (50 g, weighed out of shell), at room temperature, beaten

---

These ginger snaps are just how they sound: gingery and snappy, and somewhat spicy. You can make them dairy free by replacing the butter with an equal amount, by weight, of nonhydrogenated vegetable shortening, but they won't taste quite like the original. They'll still be delicious, but if you're going for true authenticity, make them just as written!

Preheat your oven to 325°F. Line rimmed baking sheets with unbleached parchment paper and set them aside.

In a large bowl, place the flour, cornstarch, baking soda, cinnamon, ginger, salt, and granulated sugar, and whisk to combine well. Add the brown sugar, and whisk again, working out any lumps. Create a well in the center of the dry ingredients, and add the butter, molasses, honey, vanilla, and egg, mixing to combine after each addition. The dough will be thick and smooth and somewhat sticky to the touch.

Roll out the dough between two sheets of unbleached parchment paper into a rectangle about ⅜ inch thick. If the dough seems too sticky or difficult to handle, place it in the refrigerator or freezer after you roll it out to allow it to firm up. Cut out rounds about 1¾ inches in diameter from the cookie dough. Place the rounds about 1½ inches apart from one another on the prepared baking sheets. Gather and reroll the scraps to cut out more cookies until you've used up the dough.

Place the cutouts on the baking sheets in the freezer for about 5 minutes, or until firm. Remove the baking sheets from the freezer and place, one at a time, in the center of the preheated oven and bake until the cookies are lightly golden brown and dry to the touch, about 12 minutes. Remove from the oven and allow to cool completely on the baking sheets. They will crisp as they cool.

The cookies can be stored in a sealed glass container at room temperature and should maintain their texture for at least 5 days. For longer storage, seal them tightly in a freezer-safe wrap or bag, and freeze for up to 2 months. Defrost at room temperature.

Nabisco Mallomars

MAKES ABOUT 50 COOKIES

*E*very single time I think of Mallomar cookies, I think of the movie *When Harry Met Sally*. Remember that New Year's Eve scene where Harry finally realizes that he's in love with Sally and goes off to find her at that fancy New York party? Before he takes off after her, he's watching the New Year's Eve special on television and eating Mallomars. He says to himself, "What's so bad about this? You got Dick Clark, that's tradition. You got Mallomars, the greatest cookies of all time." Make Mallomars for yourself, and you can have them again—safely gluten-free. The cookie base in this recipe is the perfect graham cracker for a Mallomar—not too hard, not too soft. To make the whole three-step process more manageable, make the cookie base ahead of time and store the cookies either in a sealed glass container at room temperature or freeze for longer storage. Then, all that's left is to make the marshmallows (which are quicker and easier than you think, as long as you have that trusty candy thermometer), pipe them on top, and allow them to set, about an hour. Then, a quick spin in some dark chocolate, and you'll swear these are actually *better* than Harry's Mallomars.

Prepare the cookies: Preheat your oven to 325°F. Line rimmed baking sheets with unbleached parchment paper and set them aside.

In a large bowl, place the flour, baking soda, baking powder, salt, and granulated sugar, and whisk to combine well. Add the brown sugar and whisk again, working out any lumps. Create a well in the center of the dry ingredients and add the shortening, golden syrup, vanilla, egg, and 2 tablespoons of the milk, mixing to combine after each addition. Knead the dough together with your hands, adding more milk, 1 teaspoonful at

---

Cookie Base

2 cups (280 g) all-purpose gluten-free flour (see page 2), plus more for sprinkling

¼ teaspoon baking soda

¼ teaspoon baking powder

⅛ teaspoon kosher salt

¼ cup (50 g) granulated sugar

⅓ cup (73 g) packed light brown sugar

6 tablespoons (70 g) nonhydrogenated vegetable shortening, melted and cooled

4 tablespoons (84 g) Lyle's golden syrup

½ teaspoon pure vanilla extract

1 egg (50 g, weighed out of shell), at room temperature, beaten

2 to 4 tablespoons (1 to 2 fluid ounces) milk, at room temperature

---

CONTINUED ON PAGE 67

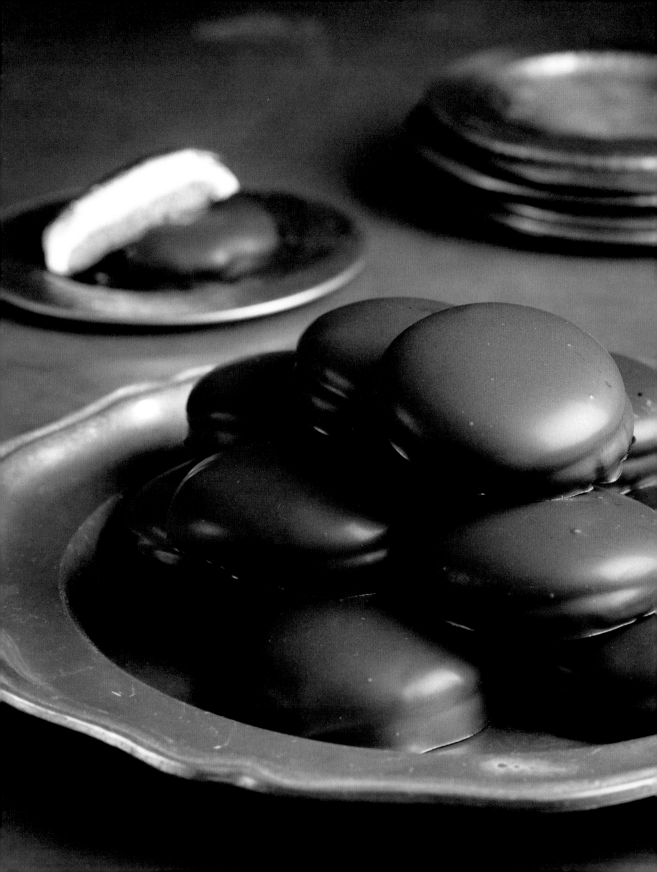

a time if necessary, to bring the dough together. Transfer the dough to a lightly floured piece of unbleached parchment paper and, sprinkling lightly with flour as necessary to prevent sticking, roll out the dough until it is about ¼ inch thick. With a floured 2-inch cookie cutter, cut out rounds and place them about 1 inch apart from one another on the prepared baking sheets. Gather and reroll the scraps to cut out more cookies until you've used up the dough. Place the baking sheets, one at a time, in the center of the preheated oven and bake until the cookies are very lightly golden brown on the edges and dry to the touch, 10 to 12 minutes. Allow the cookies to cool on the baking sheets for 5 minutes before transferring to a wire rack to cool completely.

Prepare the marshmallows: Bloom the gelatin in 2 fluid ounces (¼ cup) of the cool water by placing them together in the bowl of a stand mixer fitted with the whisk attachment, or a large bowl with a hand mixer, and mix them gently to combine. The gelatin will swell as it sits.

In a small, heavy-bottomed saucepan, place the remaining 2 ounces of cool water and the sugar and cream of tartar, and stir gently to combine. Clip a candy thermometer to the side of the saucepan, and cook over medium heat until the mixture reaches 240°F.

Pour the hot sugar mixture down the side of the mixer bowl of bloomed gelatin, whisk together with a separate, handheld whisk, and allow to cool briefly until no longer hot to the touch. Add the vanilla and salt, and beat on medium speed until the marshmallow becomes thick, white, and glossy, about 3 minutes. It should nearly triple in size. It is ready when the marshmallow mixture pours off the beaters slowly. Transfer the marshmallow to a pastry bag fitted with a ¼-inch open piping tip, and pipe mounds on top of the cooled cookies, leaving a small border around the perimeter of the cookies. Allow to sit at room temperature until the marshmallows are set, about an hour, and up to overnight.

Prepare the topping: In a medium-size, heat-safe bowl, place the chocolate and coconut oil and melt according to the instructions on page 21. Allow to cool slightly so the mixture can thicken. Turn the marshmallow-topped cookies upside down and immerse completely in the melted chocolate mixture, one at a time. Press down on the bottom of the cookie with the tines of a fork, then flip it gently in the chocolate. Pull the cookie out of the chocolate by slipping the fork under it and bobbing the cookie on the surface of the chocolate a few times before pulling it along the edge of the bowl and carefully placing it on a clean

CONTINUED FROM PAGE 65

Marshmallow Layer

¾ tablespoon (5 g) unflavored powdered gelatin

½ cup (4 fluid ounces) cool water

1 cup (200 g) granulated sugar

⅛ teaspoon cream of tartar

½ teaspoon pure vanilla extract

⅛ teaspoon kosher salt

Chocolate Topping

16 ounces dark chocolate, chopped

4 tablespoons (56 g) virgin coconut oil

sheet of waxed or parchment paper. Allow the chocolate glaze to set at room temperature.

These cookies are best enjoyed the day they are dipped in the chocolate. The finished cookies can be stored in a sealed glass container at room temperature for about 2 days. For longer storage, seal the finished cookies tightly in a freezer-safe wrap or bag, and freeze for up to 2 months. Defrost at room temperature. The chocolate coating may bloom a bit over time, but it won't affect the taste at all.

Pepperidge Farm Mint Milano Cookies

MAKES ABOUT 30 SANDWICH COOKIES

*C*rispy, chocolate-layered Milano cookies come in every flavor imaginable these days, but my heart still belongs to Mint Milanos. I'm really not sure if the Pepperidge Farm people flavor both the cookie and the filling with mint, but I went for broke and did both. And let's just say that they should really take a page out of our book, and make these tender, crunchy little sandwich cookies just like we do, with mint in the cookie, too. Art imitating life imitating art. If peppermint doesn't call your name as it does mine, try pure lemon or orange extract in its place.

Prepare the cookies: Preheat your oven to 350°F. Line rimmed baking sheets with unbleached parchment paper and set them aside.

In a small bowl, place the flour, confectioners' sugar, and salt, and whisk to combine well. Set the bowl aside.

In the bowl of a stand mixer fitted with the paddle attachment, or a large bowl with a hand mixer, place the butter and melted shortening, and beat on high speed until light and fluffy. Add the egg whites, vanilla, peppermint extract, and water, and beat until well combined. Add the dry ingredients and beat on low speed until combined. Increase the speed to medium-high and beat until smooth. Place the mixture in the refrigerator to chill for about 15 minutes, or until the consistency is thick enough to hold its shape but still pipeable. If the batter is warm, it will spread too much during baking.

Transfer the mixture to a large pastry bag fitted with a ¼-inch plain piping tip. Pipe sections of batter ¼ inch wide x 1½ inches long, about 2 inches apart from one another on the prepared baking sheet.

Place the baking sheets, one at a time, in the center of the preheated oven and bake for 8 to 10 minutes, or until the cookies are just beginning to brown around the edges. The cookies will crisp as they cool. Allow to

Cookies

1½ cups (210 g) all-purpose gluten-free flour (see page 2)

2½ cups (288 g) confectioners' sugar

⅛ teaspoon kosher salt

8 tablespoons (112 g) unsalted butter, at room temperature

4 tablespoons (48 g) nonhydrogenated vegetable shortening, melted and cooled

6 egg whites (150 g), at room temperature

1½ tablespoons pure vanilla extract

½ teaspoon pure peppermint extract

2 tablespoons (1 fluid ounce) lukewarm water

CONTINUED ON PAGE 71

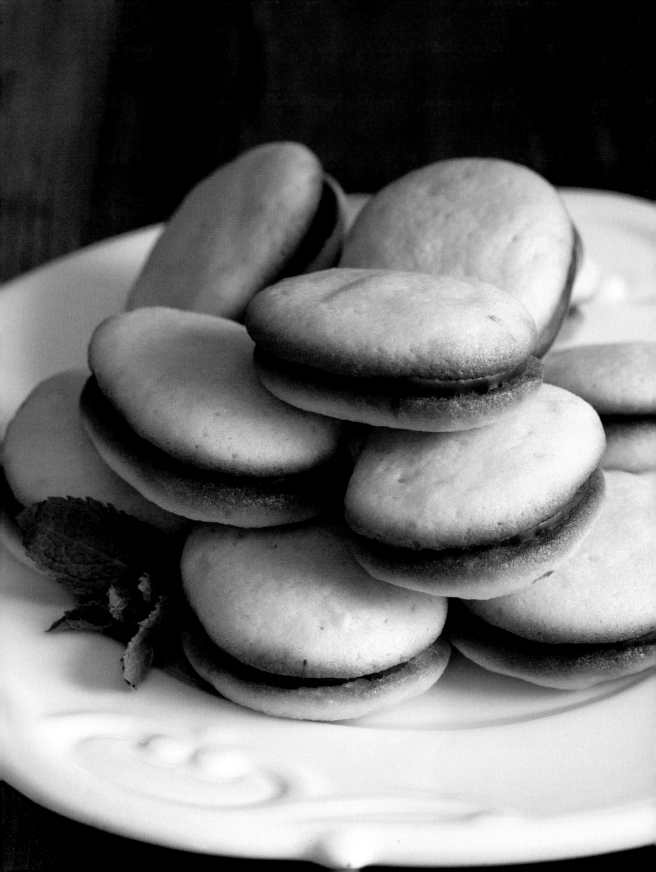

cool on the baking sheet for 5 minutes before transferring to a wire rack to cool completely.

Prepare the filling: Place the chocolate in a small, heat-safe bowl. In a small, heavy-bottomed saucepan, place the cream and heat to a simmer over medium heat. Pour the hot cream over the chocolate and allow to sit for a few minutes until the chocolate begins to melt. Add the peppermint extract and stir until smooth. Match up the most similarly shaped cookies into pairs. Invert one cookie in each pair, spoon on about 1 teaspoonful of filling, and spread into an even layer. Cover with the other cookie in the pair, right-side up, and press down gently to form a sandwich.

The finished cookies can be stored in a sealed glass container at room temperature and should maintain their texture for about 2 days. For longer storage, seal them tightly in a freezer-safe wrap or bag, and freeze for up to 2 months. Defrost at room temperature. Keep in mind that the cookies will lose some of their crispness during freezer storage.

CONTINUED FROM PAGE 69

Filling

8 ounces dark chocolate, chopped

1/2 cup (4 fluid ounces) heavy whipping cream

1/2 teaspoon pure peppermint extract

Pepperidge Farm Soft Baked Snickerdoodle Cookies

MAKES ABOUT 50 COOKIES

Cookies

2½ cups (350 g) all-purpose gluten-free flour (see page 2)

½ teaspoon kosher salt

1 teaspoon baking soda

2 teaspoons cream of tartar

1½ teaspoons ground cinnamon

1½ cups (300 g) granulated sugar

12 tablespoons (168 g) unsalted butter, at room temperature

2 eggs (100 g, weighed out of shell), at room temperature, beaten

Topping

1½ tablespoons ground cinnamon

3 tablespoons (38 g) granulated sugar

nickerdoodles: the truly lovely soft cinnamon-sugar cookie with the slightly unfortunate name. If you're like me, and you didn't grow up with snickerdoodles, the name may sound kind of silly. If you grew up with them, you might just take mild offense at my characterization. At least I hope it's mild. Cream of tartar is essential, as it gives these cookies their trademark tanginess and helps to keep them super soft and pillowy. Cream of tartar can be found in the spices section of every grocery store of any real size.

Prepare the cookies: In a large bowl, place the flour, salt, baking soda, cream of tartar, cinnamon, and sugar, and whisk to combine well. Create a well in the center of the dry ingredients, add the butter and eggs, and mix to combine. The dough should be thick but soft. Divide it equally among two large pieces of unbleached parchment paper or plastic wrap. Roll each piece in the paper or plastic into a cylinder about 1½ inches in diameter, and roll to wrap tightly, twisting the ends to seal. Place the dough in the refrigerator until firm, about 30 minutes, and up to overnight.

Prepare the topping: When you are ready to bake the cookies, place the cinnamon and sugar in a shallow bowl or on a rimmed plate, and whisk to combine well. Line rimmed baking sheets with unbleached parchment paper and set them aside. Preheat your oven to 350°F.

Remove one cylinder of dough at a time from the refrigerator. If the cylinder has lost its round shape, rock it back and forth on the counter, as if it were a rolling pin, to round out any flat edges. Slice the cylinder in cross-section into about twenty-four pieces, each about ½ inch thick. Press each disk of dough into the cinnamon-sugar topping, on both sides and on the edges if possible. Place the cinnamon-sugar-covered

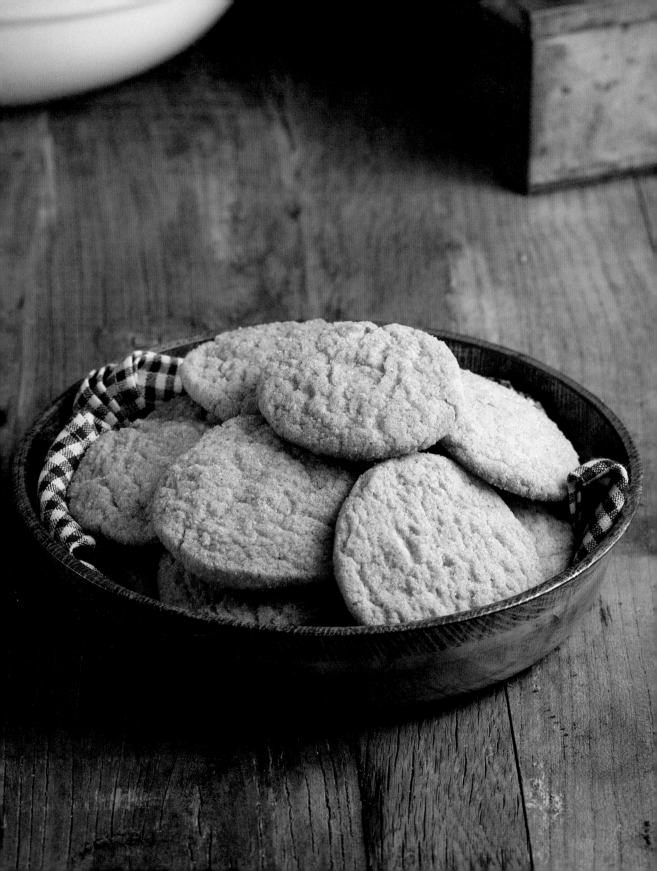

disks about 2½ inches apart on the prepared baking sheets (the cookies will spread during baking).

Place the baking sheets, one at a time, in the center of the preheated oven and bake until the cookies have spread to about double their original size, have taken upon something of a crackled appearance (as the cinnamon-sugar topping has spread), and appear set, 8 to 10 minutes. Remove from the oven and allow to cool on the baking sheets for at least 10 minutes, or until stable, before transferring to a wire rack to cool completely.

The cookies can be stored in a sealed glass container at room temperature and should maintain their texture for at least 5 days. For longer storage, seal them tightly in a freezer-safe wrap or bag, and freeze for up to 2 months. Defrost at room temperature.

Pepperidge Farm Homestyle Sugar Cookies

MAKES 15 COOKIES

These large, rustic-style, chewy sugar cookies are the sort that it's all too easy to eat one after the other. They don't weigh you down one bit, so try eating them with no distractions. Otherwise, before you know it, the whole batch is gone!

Preheat your oven to 300°F. Line rimmed baking sheets with unbleached parchment paper and set them aside.

In a large bowl, place the flour, cornstarch, baking soda, baking powder, salt, and 1 cup (200 g) of the sugar, and whisk to combine well. Create a well in the center of the dry ingredients, and add the butter, shortening, egg, and vanilla, mixing to combine after each addition. The dough will be thick and smooth but easy to shape and not greasy. If it is greasy at all, it is likely because your butter was melted, not at room temperature. Chill the dough briefly to help it firm up before proceeding with the recipe.

Place the remaining ¼ cup (50 g) of sugar in a small bowl. Divide the dough into fifteen pieces, and roll each into a ball about 1½ inches in diameter. Press each ball of dough into a disk about ¾ inch thick, and then press the disk into the remaining ¼ cup (50 g) of sugar, making sure to coat it on all sides. Place about 2 inches apart from one another on the prepared baking sheets as the cookies will spread quite a lot during baking. Place the baking sheets in the freezer to chill until firm, about 5 minutes.

Place the baking sheets, one at a time, in the center of the preheated oven and bake until the cookies are set in the center and just beginning to brown around the edges, about 12 minutes. Remove from the oven and allow to cool on the baking sheets for at least 10 minutes, or until stable, before transferring to a wire rack to cool completely.

The cookies can be stored in a sealed glass container at room temperature and should maintain their texture for at least 5 days. For longer storage, seal them tightly in a freezer-safe wrap or bag, and freeze for up to 2 months. Defrost at room temperature.

1½ cups (210 g) all-purpose gluten-free flour (see page 2)

2 tablespoons (18 g) cornstarch

½ teaspoon baking soda

¼ teaspoon baking powder

¼ teaspoon kosher salt

1¼ cups (250 g) granulated sugar, plus more for coating

6 tablespoons (84 g) unsalted butter, at room temperature

2 tablespoons (24 g) nonhydrogenated vegetable shortening, melted and cooled

1 egg (50 g, weighed out of shell), at room temperature, beaten

1 teaspoon pure vanilla extract

Pepperidge Farm Sausalito Milk Chocolate Macadamia Cookies

MAKES 16 COOKIES

4 ounces raw macadamia nut pieces

2 cups (280 g) all-purpose gluten-free flour (see page 2)

½ teaspoon baking soda

¼ teaspoon kosher salt

10 tablespoons (125 g) granulated sugar

¼ cup (55 g) packed light brown sugar

4 tablespoons (56 g) unsalted butter, at room temperature

4 tablespoons (48 g) nonhydrogenated vegetable shortening, melted and cooled

1½ teaspoons pure vanilla extract

1 egg (50 g, weighed out of shell), at room temperature, beaten

*M*acadamias are rather expensive nuts. When you buy whole nuts, you are paying a premium for that selection of only the best, roundest whole nuts. Buy a package of macadamia nut "pieces" and you'll save a bundle. These crispy Sausalito cookies pair lightly toasted macadamia nut pieces with smooth milk chocolate chips.

First, toast the nuts: Preheat your oven to 300°F. Line a rimmed baking sheet with unbleached parchment paper, and place the macadamia nut pieces on it in an even layer. Place the baking sheet in the center of the preheated oven and toast the nuts for 5 minutes. Remove the pan from the oven, shake it to redistribute the nuts, then toast them again for another 5 minutes, or until light brown and fragrant. Remove the baking sheet from the oven and set the nuts aside to cool briefly.

Raise the oven temperature to 325°F. Line the rimmed baking sheet with a clean piece of unbleached parchment paper and set aside.

In a large bowl, place the flour, baking soda, salt, and granulated sugar, and whisk to combine well. Add the brown sugar and whisk again, working out any lumps. Create a well in the center of the dry ingredients and add the butter and shortening, then the vanilla and egg, and mix to combine. The dough will be thick. Knead the dough together with your hands, adding water by the half-teaspoonful as necessary to bring the dough together. Add the chips tossed in cornstarch, and the toasted nut pieces to the cookie dough and mix until the chips are evenly distributed throughout the dough.

Place the dough on a large piece of unbleached parchment paper, and roll in the paper into a cylinder about 2½ inches in diameter. Roll to wrap tightly, twisting the ends to seal. Place the dough in the freezer until just firm, about 10 minutes.

Remove the dough from the freezer. If the cylinder of dough has lost its round shape, rock it back and forth on the counter as if it were a rolling pin to restore the round shape. Unwrap the dough and slice it with a very sharp chef's knife thickly in cross-section into rounds that are nearly ¾ inch thick. Place the rounds about 1 inch apart on the prepared baking sheet, and bake until the cookies are lightly golden brown all over and set, about 12 minutes. Allow the cookies to cool on the baking sheet for at least 10 minutes, or until stable, before transferring to a wire rack to cool completely. The cookies will crisp as they cool.

The cookies can be stored in a sealed glass container at room temperature and should maintain their texture for at least 5 days. For longer storage, seal them tightly in a freezer-safe wrap or bag, and freeze for up to 2 months. Defrost at room temperature.

Lukewarm water by the half-teaspoonful, as necessary

6 ounces milk chocolate chips, tossed in 1 teaspoon cornstarch

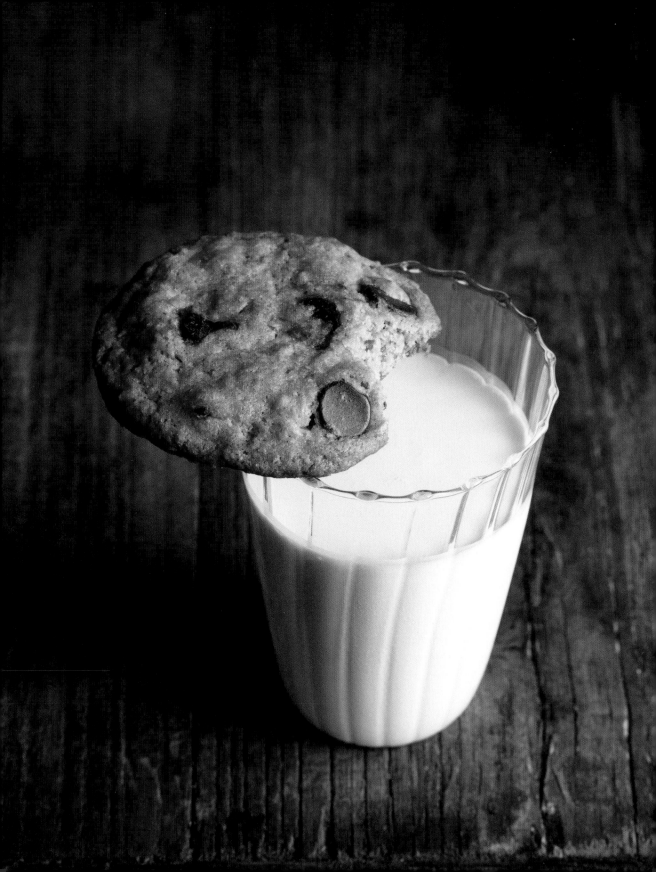

Mrs. Fields Chocolate Chip Cookies

MAKES ABOUT 24 COOKIES

*M*rs. Fields Chocolate Chip Cookies are chocolate chip cookies. They are *not* oatmeal chocolate chip cookies. Their special texture comes from the oat flour mixed with all-purpose flour (both gluten-free for us, of course). The oat flour gives these cookies a moistness and a tenderness, without making them truly soft. As always, I never purchase gluten-free oat flour as such. I simply grind certified gluten-free rolled oats in a blender or food processor as finely as possible. If you've never had the pleasure, these really taste just like the original, so now you'll know. So when you are asked that age-old question ("How do you like Mrs. Fields Chocolate Chip Cookies?"), you'll answer with authority.

Preheat your oven to 325°F. Line a rimmed baking sheet with unbleached parchment paper and set it aside.

In a large bowl, place the oat flour, all-purpose flour, baking soda, and salt, and whisk to combine well. Place the chocolate chips in a separate, medium-size bowl, add 1 tablespoon of the flour mixture, and toss the chips to coat them in the flour. Set the chips aside. To the flour mixture, add the granulated sugar and brown sugar, and whisk again to combine well, working out any lumps. Create a well in the center of the dry ingredients and add the butter, egg, and vanilla, and mix to combine. The dough will be thick. Add the floured chips to the dough, and mix until the chips are evenly distributed throughout the dough.

Drop the dough by rounded tablespoonful on the prepared baking sheet with about 1½ inches between each piece. Roll each piece of dough between slightly wet palms into a ball, and then press into a ¼-inch-thick disk. Place the baking sheet in the freezer for about 10 minutes, or until firm.

---

1 cup (120 g) certified gluten-free oat flour

1 cup (140 g) all-purpose gluten-free flour (see page 2)

¾ teaspoon baking soda

¼ teaspoon kosher salt

12 ounces semisweet chocolate chips

½ cup (100 g) granulated sugar

½ cup (109 g) packed light brown sugar

8 tablespoons (112 g) unsalted butter, at room temperature

1 egg (50 g, weighed out of shell), at room temperature, beaten

1 teaspoon pure vanilla extract

Place the baking sheet in the center of the preheated oven and bake until the cookies are lightly golden brown all over, and slightly more brown around the edges, about 9 minutes. Remove from the oven and allow to cool on the baking sheet for at least 10 minutes or until stable, before transferring to a wire rack to cool completely.

The cookies can be stored in a sealed glass container at room temperature and should maintain their texture for at least 5 days. For longer storage, seal them tightly in a freezer-safe wrap or bag, and freeze for up to 2 months. Defrost at room temperature.

Archway Soft Iced Oatmeal Cookies

MAKES ABOUT 30 COOKIES

These chewy oatmeal cookies are tender and soft and only lightly sweet. The bright white icing on top is sweeter than the cookie itself, which provides the perfect balance. I've added chocolate chips to mine, as I always knew that these were not oatmeal raisin cookies but could have sworn that I tasted chocolate chips in there. Feel free to leave them out, of course!

Prepare the cookies: Preheat your oven to 325°F. Line rimmed baking sheets with unbleached parchment paper and set them aside.

In a large bowl, place the flour, baking soda, salt, and cinnamon. Place the miniature chocolate chips in a small bowl, if using, and add 1 teaspoon of the dry ingredients and toss to coat. Set the chips aside. To the large bowl of dry ingredients, add the granulated sugar and brown sugar, and whisk to combine well, working out any lumps. Add the rolled oats, and mix to combine well. Create a well in the center of the dry ingredients and add the butter, shortening, egg, egg yolk, and vanilla, and mix to combine. Add the floured chocolate chips and mix until the chips are evenly distributed throughout. The dough will be sticky.

Drop the dough by rounded tablespoonful, about 1½ inches apart, on the prepared baking sheets. With wet fingers, press each piece of dough into a disk about ¼ inch high.

Place the baking sheets, one at a time, in the center of the preheated oven and bake until the cookies are lightly brown around the edges and set in the center, about 7 minutes. Allow to cool on the baking sheets for at least 10 minutes, or until stable, before transferring to a wire rack to cool completely.

While the cookies are cooling, prepare the icing: In a medium-size bowl, place the confectioners' sugar. Add the lemon juice and 1 tablespoon of the water, and mix to form a very thick paste. Add another tablespoon of water, or more if necessary, and mix until smooth and well combined. The icing should be opaque but thickly pourable.

Cookies

¾ cup (105 g) all-purpose gluten-free flour (see page 2)

½ teaspoon baking soda

¼ teaspoon kosher salt

¼ teaspoon ground cinnamon

4 ounces miniature chocolate chips (optional)

3 tablespoons (38 g) granulated sugar

½ cup (109 g) packed light brown sugar

1½ cups (150 g) certified gluten-free old-fashioned rolled oats

4 tablespoons (56 g) unsalted butter, at room temperature

4 tablespoons (48 g) nonhydrogenated vegetable shortening, melted and cooled

CONTINUED ON PAGE 83

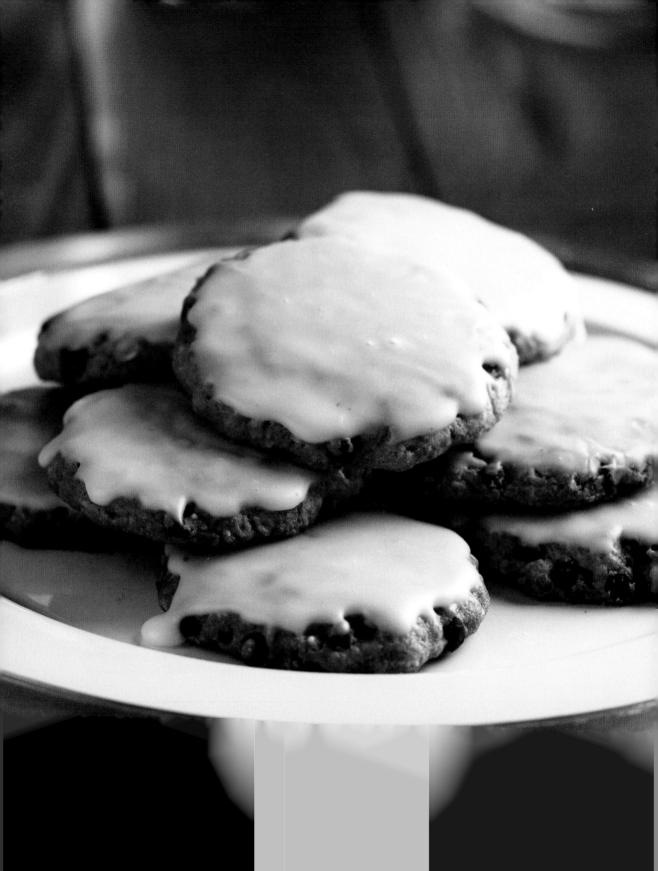

Place a sheet of parchment or waxed paper underneath the wire rack on which the cookies are resting. Once the cookies are cool, spoon about 1 tablespoon of icing on top of each of the cookies. Allow to set and harden at room temperature.

The cookies can be stored in a sealed glass container at room temperature and should maintain their texture for at least 5 days. For longer storage, seal them tightly in a freezer-safe wrap or bag, and freeze for up to 2 months. Defrost at room temperature.

CONTINUED FROM PAGE 81

1 egg (50 g, weighed out of shell) plus 1 egg yolk (25 g), at room temperature, beaten

1 teaspoon pure vanilla extract

Icing

2 cups (230 g) confectioners' sugar

1 teaspoon (½ fluid ounce) freshly squeezed lemon juice

2 to 3 tablespoons lukewarm water (1 to 1½ fluid ounce), plus more by the quarter-teaspoonful if necessary

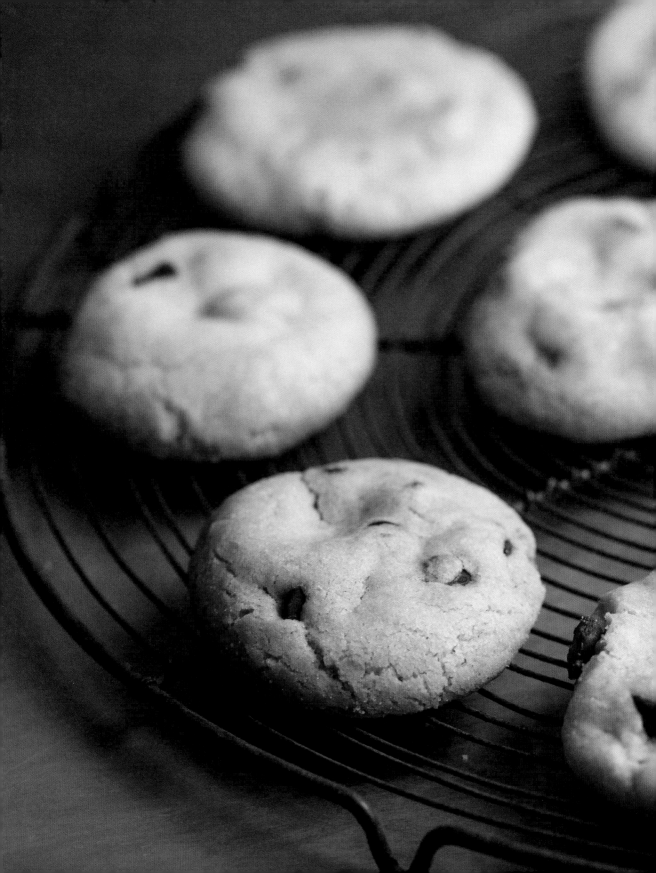

Keebler Soft Batch Chocolate Chip Cookies

MAKES 20 COOKIES

Soft-batch cookies are meant to taste as if they just came out of the oven; problem is, when cookies have just come out of the oven, if you try to eat them, they'll fall apart and make a terrible mess. These cookies are *better* than that: soft and chewy but easy to eat, and stay neat and clean. They are made with gluten-free cake flour for the perfect soft texture. As with the other recipes in this book, make ingredient substitutions at your own risk. Only the precise balance of ingredients in the list below, with the method described, will yield the tender results we seek.

Preheat your oven to 325°F. Line rimmed baking sheets with unbleached parchment paper and set them aside.

In a large bowl, place the cake flour, salt, baking soda, and granulated sugar, and whisk to combine well. Add the brown sugar, and whisk again to combine, working out any lumps. Create a well in the center of the dry ingredients, and add the butter, shortening, vanilla, egg, and egg yolk, mixing to combine well after each addition. The dough will be thick and soft. Add the cornstarch-dusted chips, and mix until evenly distributed throughout the dough.

Divide the dough into pieces of about 2½ tablespoons each, roll each tightly into a ball between your palms, and then place about 2 inches apart on the prepared baking sheets. Flatten the balls of dough slightly into disks about ¾ inch thick. Place the baking sheets in the freezer to chill for about 10 minutes, or until firm.

Once the dough has chilled, place the baking sheets, one at a time, in the center of the preheated oven and bake just until the balls of dough have melted and spread and the cookies are set in the center, about 12 minutes. They will be very lightly browned around the edges, and some may even be slightly wet toward the center. Be careful not to

2¼ cups (315 g) gluten-free cake flour (see page 2)

½ teaspoon kosher salt

1 teaspoon baking soda

⅔ cup (133 g) granulated sugar

½ cup (109 g) packed light brown sugar

6 tablespoons (84 g) unsalted butter, at room temperature

5 tablespoons (60 g) nonhydrogenated vegetable shortening, melted and cooled

1 tablespoon pure vanilla extract

1 egg (50 g, weighed out of shell) plus 1 egg yolk (25 g), at room temperature, beaten

1 cup (6 ounces) semisweet chocolate chips, tossed with 1 teaspoon cornstarch

overbake them. Remove from the oven and allow to cool on the baking sheets for at least 10 minutes, or until stable, before transferring to a wire rack to cool completely.

The cookies can be stored in a sealed glass container at room temperature and should maintain their texture for at least 5 days. For longer storage, seal them tightly in a freezer-safe wrap or bag, and freeze for up to 2 months. Defrost at room temperature.

Keebler Fudge Stripes Cookies, Original

MAKES ABOUT 35 COOKIES

You'd think that a simple shortbread cookie with a thin layer of chocolate on the bottom and stripes across the top would taste just the same as if you, say, ate a shortbread cookie and a piece of chocolate at the same time. Well, I tried that in the name of science, and I can report with confidence that it is *not* the same as eating one of these Fudge Stripes–style cookies at *all*. Eating brand-name snacks isn't just about the ingredients. It's about the whole experience. And if you want to experience fudge stripe cookies as you remember them to be, you'd better get dipping and drizzling that chocolate.

Prepare the cookies: Preheat your oven to 350°F. Line rimmed baking sheets with unbleached parchment paper and set them aside.

In a large bowl, place the flour, nonfat dry milk, and salt, and whisk to combine well. Create a well in the center of the dry ingredients and add the butter, golden syrup, and 2 tablespoons of the water, mixing to combine after each addition. Knead with your hands to bring the dough together, adding more water by the half-teaspoonful as necessary.

Transfer the dough to a large piece of unbleached parchment paper and roll out until it is ¼ inch thick, sprinkling lightly with flour as necessary to prevent sticking. Cut out rounds with a 2½-inch cookie cutter, and cut a ¾-inch hole in the center of each. Place the cookies about 1 inch apart from one another on the prepared baking sheets. Gather and reroll the scraps to cut out more cookies until you've used up the dough.

Place the baking sheets, one at a time, in the center of the preheated oven and bake until the cookies are lightly golden brown all over, about 12 minutes. Allow to cool on the baking sheets for 5 minutes before transferring to a wire rack to cool completely.

While the cookies are cooling, prepare the glaze: Line another rimmed baking sheet with a piece of parchment or waxed paper and set it aside.

Cookies

1¾ cups (245 g) all-purpose gluten-free flour (see page 2), plus more for sprinkling

3 tablespoons plus 1 teaspoon (20 g) nonfat dry milk, ground into a finer powder

⅛ teaspoon kosher salt

8 tablespoons (112 g) unsalted butter, at room temperature

2 tablespoons (42 g) Lyle's golden syrup

2 to 4 tablespoons (1 to 2 fluid ounces) lukewarm water

Chocolate Glaze

8 ounces semisweet chocolate, chopped

2 tablespoons (28 g) virgin coconut oil

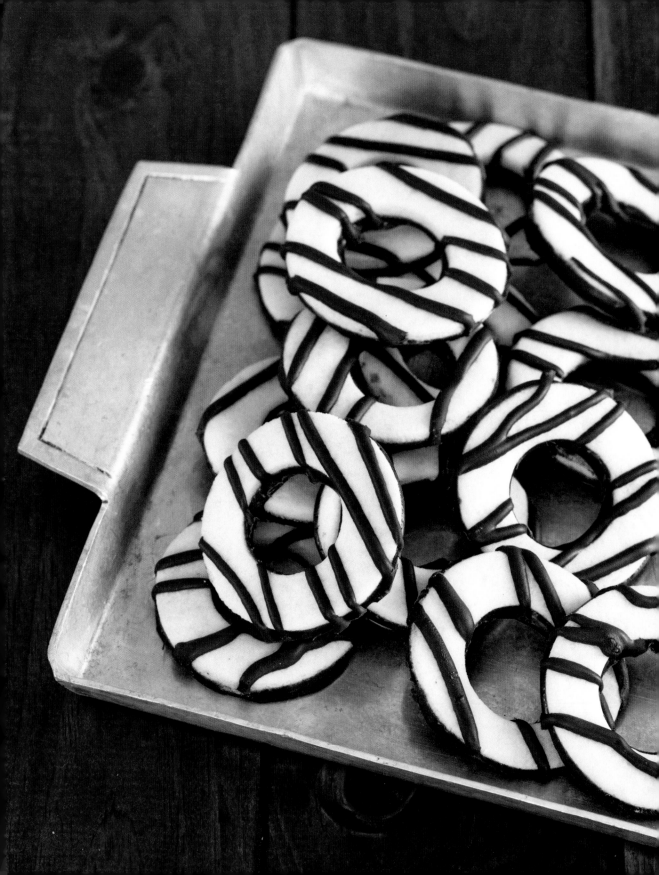

In a medium-size, heat-safe bowl, place the chocolate and coconut oil and melt according to the instructions on page 21. Cool slightly to allow the mixture to begin to thicken. Dip the bottoms of all the cookies in the chocolate, and place them chocolate side down on the lined baking sheet. Transfer the remaining chocolate to a pastry bag fitted with a very small open piping tip (a #2 tip works great) and pipe stripes on top of each cookie. Allow the cookies to sit at room temperature until set.

The cookies can be stored in a sealed glass container at room temperature and should maintain their texture for at least 5 days. For longer storage, seal the plain shortbread cookies tightly in a freezer-safe wrap or bag, and freeze for up to 2 months. Defrost at room temperature before dipping in and striping with chocolate.

Keebler Sandies Pecan Shortbread Cookies

MAKES 16 COOKIES

1¾ cups (245 g) all-purpose gluten-free flour (see page 2)

¼ teaspoon baking soda

⅛ teaspoon kosher salt

3 tablespoons plus 1 teaspoon (20 g) nonfat dry milk, ground into a finer powder

¾ cup (150 g) granulated sugar

8 tablespoons (112 g) unsalted butter, at room temperature

1 egg yolk (25 g), at room temperature

2 to 4 tablespoons (1 to 2 fluid ounces) lukewarm water

3 ounces chopped raw or toasted pecans tossed with 1 teaspoon cornstarch

The classic Keebler Sandies variety, these crunchy short-bread cookies call for soft and tender raw pecans. But because the pecans are a mix-in, you can dress the cookies up however you like. Try using roasted or even candied pecans instead, for a twist. These are the perfect cookie for when you're in the mood for something sweet but not too sweet. Be sure to let them cool on the baking sheet for the full 10 minutes as directed in the recipe, or they'll crumble. Once cool, they're as stable as could be.

Preheat your oven to 325°F. Line a rimmed baking sheet with un-bleached parchment paper and set it aside.

In a large bowl, place the flour, baking soda, salt, nonfat dry milk, and sugar, and whisk to combine well. Create a well in the center of the dry ingredients, and add the butter, egg yolk, and 2 tablespoons of the water, mixing to combine after each addition. Add the cornstarch-dusted pe-cans and mix until evenly distributed through the dough. Knead with your hands to bring the dough together well, adding more water by the half-teaspoonful as necessary. Place the dough on a large piece of un-bleached parchment paper and roll into a log 2 inches in diameter. Wrap tightly into a cylinder, and place in the refrigerator to chill for about 10 minutes, or until firm enough to slice. Remove from the refrigerator, unwrap the dough, and slice by cross-section into ¾-inch-thick disks. Place 1 inch apart from one another on the prepared baking sheet.

Place the baking sheet in the center of the preheated oven and bake for 19 to 21 minutes, or until the cookies are light golden brown and dry to the touch. Allow to cool on the baking sheet for 10 minutes before transferring to a wire rack to cool completely.

Once cool, these cookies can be stored in a sealed glass container at room temperature and should maintain their texture for at least 5 days. For longer storage, seal the cookies tightly in a freezer-safe wrap or bag, and freeze for up to 2 months. Defrost at room temperature.

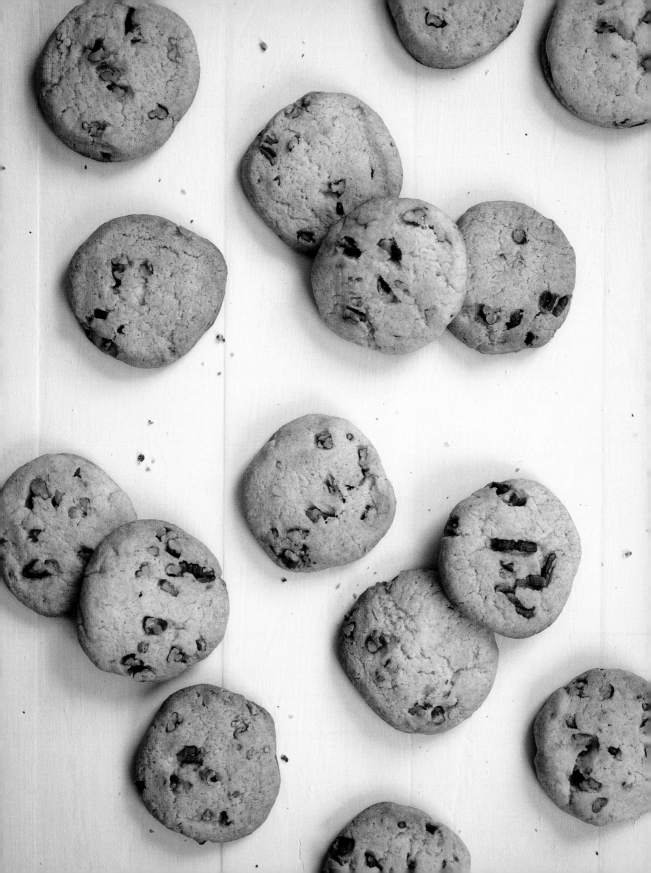

Keebler Sandies Dark Chocolate Almond Shortbread Cookies

MAKES 16 COOKIES

1¾ cups (245 g) all-purpose gluten-free flour (see page 2)

¼ teaspoon baking soda

⅛ teaspoon kosher salt

3 tablespoons plus 1 teaspoon (20 g) nonfat dry milk, ground into a finer powder

¾ cup (150 g) granulated sugar

8 tablespoons (112 g) unsalted butter, at room temperature

1 egg yolk (25 g), at room temperature

2 to 4 tablespoons (1 to 2 fluid ounces) lukewarm water

3 ounces dark chocolate chips, tossed with ½ teaspoon cornstarch

2 ounces chopped raw almonds, tossed with ½ teaspoon cornstarch

*L*ike their pecan cousins, these Sandies shortbread–style cookies melt in your mouth. This time, rich dark chocolate and crunchy almond pieces take center stage. Unlike in the pecan shortbread cookies recipe, I wouldn't recommend toasting the nuts here, as almonds aren't as soft and tender as pecans.

Preheat your oven to 325°F. Line a rimmed baking sheet with unbleached parchment paper and set it aside.

In a large bowl, place the flour, baking soda, salt, nonfat dry milk, and sugar, and whisk to combine well. Create a well in the center of the dry ingredients, and add the butter, egg yolk, and 2 tablespoons of the water, mixing to combine after each addition. Add the cornstarch-dusted chocolate chips and almonds, and mix until evenly distributed through the dough. Knead with your hands to bring the dough together well, adding more water by the half-teaspoonful as necessary. Place the dough on a large piece of unbleached parchment paper and roll into a log 2 inches in diameter. Wrap tightly into a cylinder, and place in the refrigerator to chill for about 10 minutes, or until firm enough to slice. Remove from the refrigerator, unwrap the dough, and slice by cross-section into ¾-inch-thick disks. Place 1 inch apart from one another on the prepared baking sheet.

Place the baking sheet in the center of the preheated oven and bake for 19 to 21 minutes, or until the cookies are light golden brown and dry to the touch. Allow to cool on the baking sheet for 10 minutes before transferring to a wire rack to cool completely.

Once cool, these cookies can be stored in a sealed glass container at room temperature and should maintain their texture for at least 5 days. For longer storage, seal the cookies tightly in a freezer-safe wrap or bag, and freeze for up to 2 months. Defrost at room temperature.

Keebler Vienna Fingers Creme Filled Sandwich Cookies

MAKES ABOUT 20 SANDWICH COOKIES

Remember Vienna Fingers? In case you think they're just like Golden Oreos (page 56), allow me to refresh your cookie recollection. Golden Oreos are crunchy, and the cookie part sticks in your teeth (not a judgment, just an observation). Vienna Fingers are melt-in-your-mouth-tender cookies, like a cross between butter cookies and vanilla wafers. Same filling, quite the different cookie: Whereas our Golden Oreo recipe calls for all-purpose gluten-free flour blend, here we achieve a delicate texture with gluten-free cake flour and confectioners' sugar. Each has its place in our cookie repertoire.

Prepare the cookies: Preheat your oven to 350°F. Line rimmed baking sheets with unbleached parchment paper and set them aside.

In a large bowl, place the cake flour, confectioners' sugar, and salt, and whisk to combine well. Create a well in the center of the dry ingredients and add the butter and egg, and mix to combine. Knead the dough with your hands, adding water by the half-teaspoonful if necessary to bring the dough together.

Place the dough between two sheets of unbleached parchment paper and roll it into a rectangle a bit less than ¼ inch thick. Place the rolled-out dough in the freezer to chill for 5 minutes, or until firm. Take the dough out of the freezer, remove the top sheet of paper, and cut out shapes with an oval cookie cutter about 2½ inches long. Place the shapes about 1 inch apart from one another on the prepared baking sheets. Gather and reroll the scraps to cut out more cookies until you've used up the dough.

Place the baking sheets, one at a time, in the center of the preheated oven and bake until the cookies are just beginning to brown on the

Cookies

1½ cups (210 g) gluten-free cake flour (see page 2)

½ cup (58 g) confectioners' sugar

¼ teaspoon kosher salt

8 tablespoons (112 g) unsalted butter, at room temperature

1 egg (50 g, weighed out of shell), at room temperature, beaten

Lukewarm water by the half-teaspoonful, as necessary

Filling

Stiff Sandwich Cookie Filling (page 109)

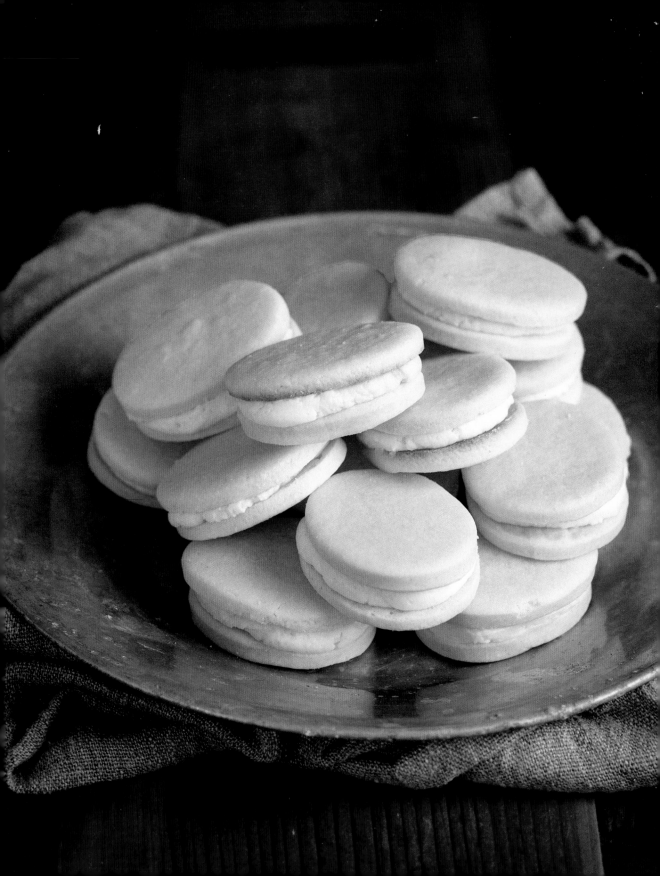

edges, about 10 minutes. Remove from the oven and allow to cool on the baking sheets for 10 minutes before transferring to a wire rack to cool completely.

Once the cookies are nearly cool, prepare the Stiff Sandwich Cookie Filling. Transfer the filling to a pastry bag fitted with a ½-inch open piping tip and invert half of the cookies. Pipe about 1 tablespoon of filling on the inverted, cooled wafer cookies. Top with the other cookies and push down gently to form a sandwich.

The filled cookies can be stored in a sealed glass container at room temperature and should maintain their texture for at least 5 days. For longer storage, seal the unfilled vanilla wafers tightly in a freezer-safe wrap or bag, and freeze for up to 2 months. Defrost at room temperature and fill as directed.

Keebler Simply Made Butter Cookies

MAKES ABOUT 30 COOKIES

1½ cups (210 g) all-purpose gluten-free flour (see page 2)

10 tablespoons (72 g) confectioners' sugar

¼ teaspoon kosher salt

8 tablespoons (112 g) unsalted butter, at room temperature

3 egg yolks (75 g), at room temperature

1 teaspoon pure vanilla extract

Lukewarm water by the half-teaspoonful, as necessary

*K*eebler's "Simply Made" line of cookies has fewer ingredients than most packaged cookies. They're made, well, from simple ingredients. Every recipe in this book began from the list of ingredients on the manufacturer's package, so these basic butter cookies made my job *much* easier. Cheers for simplicity! These cookies are lighter and more tender than traditional butter cookies, almost like a buttery sugar cookie. They're perfect for when you just want a little something with your afternoon tea.

Preheat your oven to 350°F. Line rimmed baking sheets with unbleached parchment paper and set them aside.

In a large bowl, place the flour, confectioners' sugar, and salt, and whisk to combine well. Create a well in the center of the dry ingredients, and add the butter, egg yolks, and vanilla, mixing to combine after each addition. Knead the dough until it holds together easily, adding water by the half-teaspoonful as necessary. Transfer the dough to a piece of plastic wrap, and shape it into a cylinder about 2 inches in diameter. Slice the room-temperature dough into cross-section pieces a bit more than ¼ inch wide. Place the cookies about 2 inches apart from one another on the prepared baking sheets.

Place the baking sheets, one at a time, in the center of the preheated oven and bake until the cookies are just beginning to turn lightly brown around the edges, about 8 minutes. Cool completely on the baking sheets to allow the cookies to set and become stable.

The cookies can be stored in a sealed glass container at room temperature and should maintain their texture for at least 5 days. For longer storage, seal them tightly in a freezer-safe wrap or bag, and freeze for up to 2 months. Defrost at room temperature.

Lotus Biscoff Cookies

MAKES ABOUT 50 COOKIES

*T*hey say that Biscoff cookies, also known as Speculoos, are "Europe's favorite cookie with coffee." I can't judge that favoritism independently, living in the United States as I do. But I can tell you that these crisp, caramelized-sugar cookies are really nice with a cup of coffee. I was a woman obsessed with finding just the right 2½-inch-long rectangular cookie cutter with rounded edges to make the proper Biscoff cookie shape, but finally I gave up and made my own with a Make Your Own Cookie Cutter kit. In defense of my frivolity, we were taking photos of my cookies. If you're baking for yourself, friends, and family, and you don't need the cookies to be just so, I'd go with a straight-up rectangle.

Preheat your oven to 350°F. Line rimmed baking sheets with unbleached parchment paper and set them aside.

In a large bowl, place the flour, cinnamon, salt, baking soda, and granulated sugar, and whisk to combine well. Add the brown sugar, and whisk again, working to break up any lumps. Create a well in the center of the dry ingredients, and add the butter and water, mixing to combine. Knead with your hands to bring the dough together.

Divide the dough into two equal portions and roll each between two sheets of unbleached parchment paper into a rectangle between ⅛ and ¼ inch thick. Place the rolled-out dough on a baking sheet or cutting board and place in the freezer until firm but not frozen, about 10 minutes. Remove from the freezer and cut out 2½ x ¾-inch rectangles, placing them about 1 inch apart from one another on the prepared baking sheets. Gather and reroll the scraps to cut out more cookies until you've used up the dough.

Place the baking sheets, one at a time, in the center of the preheated oven and bake until the cookies are golden brown and mostly firm to

---

2 cups (280 g) all-purpose gluten-free flour (see page 2)

1 tablespoon ground cinnamon

¼ teaspoon kosher salt

¾ teaspoon baking soda

½ cup (100 g) granulated sugar

½ cup (109 g) packed light brown sugar

8 tablespoons (112 g) unsalted butter, at room temperature

¼ cup (2 fluid ounces) water, at room temperature

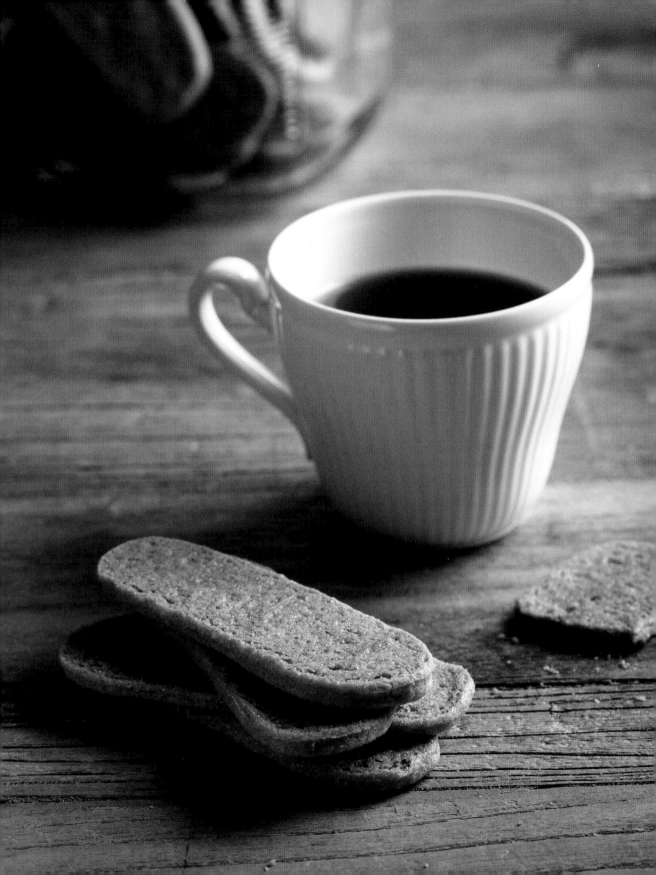

the touch, about 10 minutes. Allow the cookies to cool for 5 minutes on the baking sheets before transferring to a wire rack to cool completely. They will crisp as they cool. Serve the cookies bottom-side up, as the underside is smooth and a bit more beautiful than the top of the cookies.

The cookies can be stored in a sealed glass container at room temperature and should maintain their texture for at least 5 days. For longer storage, seal them tightly in a freezer-safe wrap or bag, and freeze for up to 2 months. Defrost at room temperature.

Lofthouse Sugar Cookies

MAKES ABOUT 30 COOKIES

Cookies

2 cups (280 g) all-purpose gluten-free flour (see page 2)

¾ teaspoon baking powder

¼ teaspoon kosher salt

½ cup (100 g) granulated sugar

3 tablespoons (22 g) confectioners' sugar

8 tablespoons (112 g) unsalted butter, at room temperature

1 egg (50 g, weighed out of shell), at room temperature, beaten

½ teaspoon pure vanilla extract

Lukewarm water by the half-teaspoonful, as necessary

For Decoration

Stiff Sandwich Cookie Filling (page 109)

Clear or multicolored sprinkles (optional)

*L*ofthouse Sugar Cookies are the big, soft, sweet cookies with a thick layer of frosting—and lots of sprinkles. They're like that eccentric aunt or cousin in the family who has an outfit for every occasion and holiday, some getups more tasteful than others. It's Halloween? She'll dress in orange, perhaps with pumpkin stripes. It's Christmas? Break out the red and green sweater! She might seem a little silly sometimes, but you have to admire the effort. And if she were these cookies, she'd also taste tender and delicious. These are, hands down, the perfect cut-out sugar cookies. Dress them up by the holiday or stick with simple rounds, decked in white— a classic.

Prepare the cookies: Preheat your oven to 350°F. Line rimmed baking sheets with unbleached parchment paper and set them aside.

In a large bowl, place the flour, baking powder, salt, granulated sugar, and confectioners' sugar, and whisk to combine well. Create a well in the center of the dry ingredients and add the butter, egg, and vanilla, and mix to combine. Knead the dough with your hands, adding water by the half-teaspoonful as necessary to bring it together. Roll the dough between two sheets of unbleached parchment paper until it is a bit less than ⅓ inch thick. Using a 2½-inch round cookie cutter, cut out rounds of dough and place them about 1 inch apart from one another on the prepared baking sheets. Gather and reroll the scraps to cut out more cookies until you've used up the dough.

Place the baking sheets, one at a time, in the center of the preheated oven and bake until the cookies are just set, about 6 minutes. The edges of some of the cookies may brown slightly, but take them out before there is any significant browning. Allow the cookies to cool on the baking sheets for 5 minutes before transferring to a wire rack to cool completely.

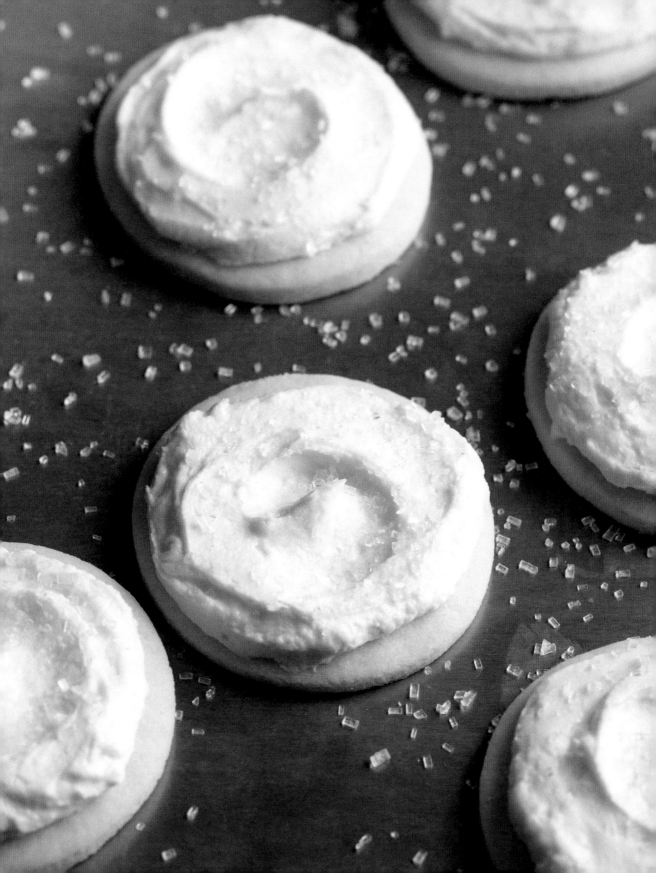

Decorate the cookies: Prepare the Stiff Sandwich Cookie Filling. Once the cookies are completely cool, spoon a generous amount of the filling onto the top of each, to serve as frosting, and spread it into an even layer with a wide knife or offset spatula. Scatter sprinkles on top, if desired. Allow to set at room temperature until the frosting hardens a bit.

The frosted cookies can be stored in a sealed plastic or glass container in the refrigerator and should maintain their texture for about 3 days. For longer storage, seal the unfrosted cookies tightly in a freezer-safe wrap or bag, and freeze for up to 2 months. Defrost at room temperature and frost and decorate as directed.

Little Debbie Star Crunch

MAKES 20 COOKIES

I don't mean to brag, but if you look online for a copycat version of Little Debbie Star Crunch cookies, you'll mostly just find chocolate crispy rice marshmallow treats with some added caramel. That's just not right. Star Crunch cookies have an actual *cookie* in the center. It's very thin and quite chewy, and it sits in the very center, surrounded on all sides by chocolate crisp rice cereal held together with sweet, gooey caramel. If you've never had a Little Debbie Star Crunch, you are about to find out what you've been missing. If you have, you *know* what I'm talkin' about.

Prepare the cookies: Preheat your oven to 325°F. Line rimmed baking sheets with unbleached parchment paper and set them aside.

In a large bowl, place the flour, cocoa powder, baking soda, salt, and granulated sugar, and whisk to combine well. Add the brown sugar and oats and mix to combine, working out any lumps. Create a well in the center of the dry ingredients and add the shortening, egg, egg yolk, and vanilla, and mix to combine. Knead the dough with your hands. It will be sticky.

Place the dough between two sheets of unbleached parchment paper and roll out into a rectangle about ⅛ inch thick. Chill the dough so that it is easier to handle. Remove the top sheet of paper and cut out rounds using a 2-inch cookie cutter. Gather and reroll the scraps to cut out more cookies until you've used up the dough. If at any point the dough becomes too difficult to handle, place it in the freezer to firm up a bit. Place the rounds of dough about 1 inch apart on the prepared baking sheets and place, one at a time, in the center of the oven. Bake for 7 minutes, or until just beginning to brown on the edges. Allow to cool to room temperature and then place in the freezer until firm, about 5 minutes. That will make them much easier to coat.

Cookies

¾ cup (105 g) all-purpose gluten-free flour (see page 2)

2 tablespoons (10 g) unsweetened cocoa powder

½ teaspoon baking soda

¼ teaspoon kosher salt

2 tablespoons (25 g) granulated sugar

½ cup (109 g) packed light brown sugar

1 cup (100 g) certified gluten-free old-fashioned rolled oats

6 tablespoons (72 g) nonhydrogenated vegetable shortening, melted and cooled

1 egg (50 g, weighed out of shell) plus 1 egg yolk (25 g), at room temperature, beaten

1 teaspoon pure vanilla extract

CONTINUED ON PAGE 104

CONTINUED FROM PAGE 103

Chocolate Caramel Crisp Rice Layer

3 cups (90 g) gluten-free crisp rice cereal

2 tablespoons (10 g) unsweetened cocoa powder

1 cup Soft Caramel for Candies (page 291), chopped

2 tablespoons (1 fluid ounce) milk

1 tablespoon (14 g) unsalted butter

4 ounces milk chocolate, chopped

Prepare the crisp rice layer: In a large bowl, place the rice cereal and cocoa powder, and toss to coat the cereal in the cocoa. Set the bowl aside. In a medium, heavy-bottomed saucepan, place the chopped caramel, milk, butter, and chocolate. Place over medium heat and heat, stirring frequently, until melted and smooth, about 4 minutes. Remove from the heat and allow the mixture to cool until no longer hot to the touch. Scrape into the bowl of cocoa-dusted rice cereal and mix gently to combine. If you add the rice cereal while the chocolate caramel mixture is still hot, the cereal tends to taste as if it has become stale, no matter how fresh it is. Remove the cookies from the freezer and immerse them, one at a time, in the rice mixture. Remove from the rice mixture with a chocolate-dipping tool or large fork, scrape along the side of the dipping bowl to brush off excess, and place on a large piece of waxed or parchment paper. Allow to set at room temperature.

These are best enjoyed the day they are dipped in the chocolate coating or the following day. For longer storage, seal the cookies tightly in a freezer-safe wrap or bag and freeze for up to 2 months. Defrost at room temperature and continue with the instructions for the crisp rice layer.

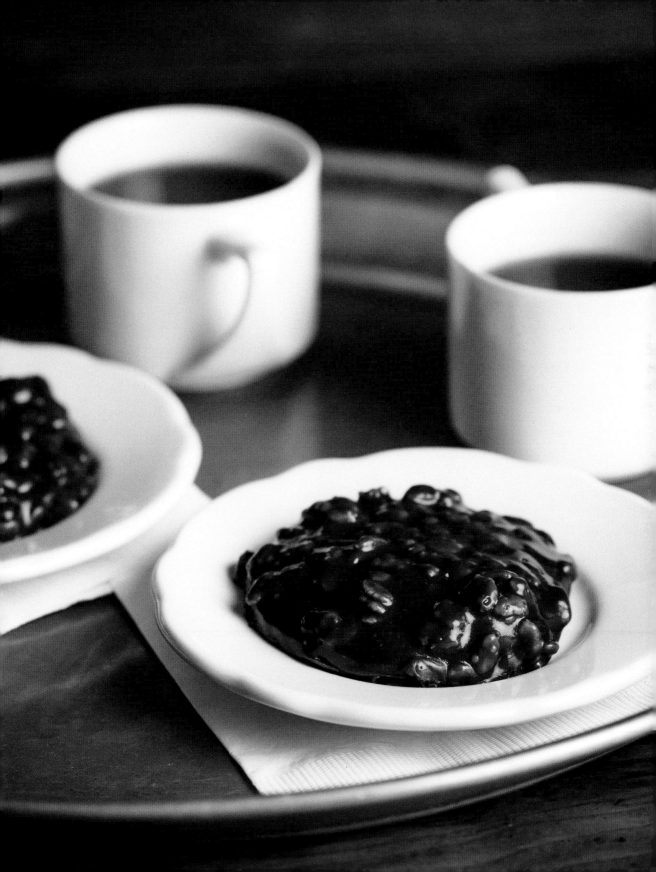

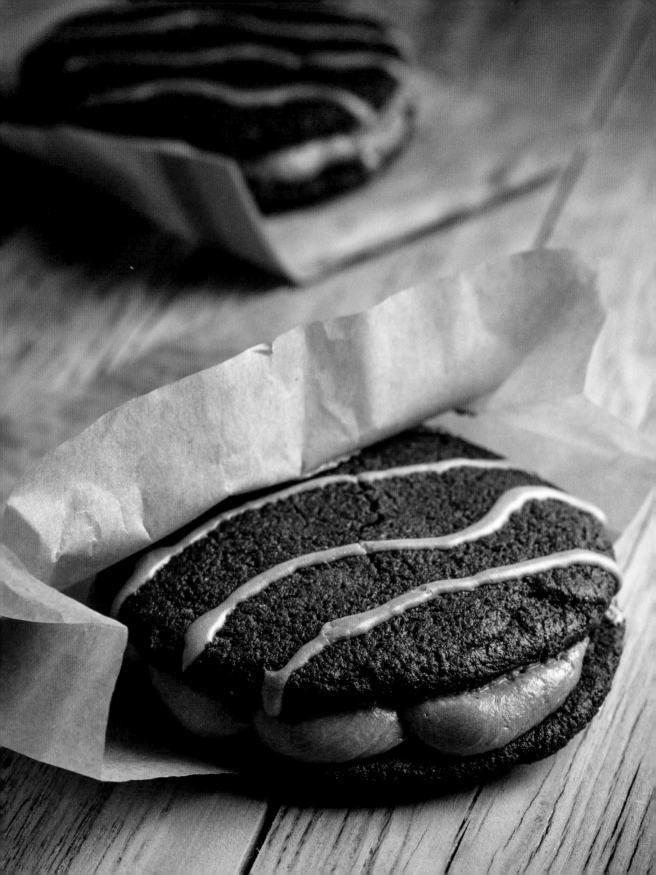

Little Debbie Fudge Rounds

MAKES 12 SANDWICH COOKIES

*J*f you're planning to pack these rich, chocolaty Little Debbie Fudge Rounds sandwich cookies in a lucky child's lunchbox (or the lunchbox of your lucky grown-up partner), I'd recommend increasing the baking time by about 3 minutes to make for a slightly crisp, more stable cookie. Otherwise, the soft chocolate cookies have a tendency to break in transit. By the time they're ready to dig in to lunch, the chocolate filling will have softened the cookies just enough to leave your loved one with the perfect indulgent lunchtime treat. These deep chocolate cookies are almost as rich as brownies, and the creamy chocolate filling is firm enough to hold up big bites.

Prepare the cookies: Preheat your oven to 325°F. Line rimmed baking sheets with unbleached parchment paper and set them aside.

In a medium-size, heat-safe bowl, melt the chopped chocolate with the chopped butter according to the instructions on page 21. Add the molasses, vanilla, and brown sugar, and mix to combine. Set the bowl aside.

In a large bowl, place the flour, cocoa powder, salt, and baking soda, and whisk to combine well. Create a well in the center of the dry ingredients, and add the melted chocolate mixture, and then the egg and egg yolk, mixing to combine after each addition. Divide the dough into twenty-four equal pieces, each about 2 ½ tablespoons. Roll each piece of dough into a round between wet palms, press into a disk about ¼ inch tall, and place about 2 inches apart on the prepared baking sheets. Place the baking sheets, one at a time, in the center of the preheated oven and bake until each cookie has spread to about 3 inches in diameter and is set in the center, about 12 minutes. Cool completely on the baking sheets.

Prepare the Chocolate Stiff Sandwich Cookie Filling. On a flat, parchment- or waxed paper–lined surface, match up the cooled cookies

Cookies

4 ounces bittersweet chocolate, chopped

8 tablespoons (112 g) unsalted butter, chopped

2 tablespoons (42 g) unsulfured molasses

1 teaspoon pure vanilla extract

⅔ cup (145 g) packed light brown sugar

1¼ cups (175 g) all-purpose gluten-free flour (see page 2)

2 tablespoons (10 g) unsweetened cocoa powder

½ teaspoon kosher salt

¼ teaspoon baking soda

1 egg (50 g, weighed out of shell) plus 1 egg yolk (25 g), at room temperature, beaten

CONTINUED ON NEXT PAGE

CONTINUED FROM PAGE 107

Filling

**Stiff Sandwich Cookie
Filling, Chocolate
Variation (page 109)**

Warm water, as needed

into pairs, and invert one cookie from each pair. Transfer most of the filling to a large pastry bag fitted with a ½-inch plain piping tip, and, on the inverted cookies, pipe about 2 tablespoons of filling. Top with the other cookie of the pair, right-side up, and press down gently to form a sandwich. Add a bit of warm water to the remaining filling to thin it a bit, and transfer the filling to a small pastry bag fitted with a very small plain piping tip (a #2 tip works well) and pipe stripes of filling on top of each cookie sandwich. Allow to set at room temperature.

The filled cookies can be stored in a sealed glass or plastic container at room temperature and should maintain their texture for about 2 days. For longer storage, seal the unfilled cookies tightly in a freezer-safe wrap or bag, and freeze for up to 2 months. Defrost at room temperature and fill as directed.

Stiff Sandwich Cookie Filling

MAKES ABOUT 2 CUPS FILLING

*T*his is the filling that you use when you want to be able to sandwich it between two cookies (such as Oreos, pages 53–58), or pile it on top of a soft sugar cookie (such as Lofthouse Sugar Cookies, page 100) and have it set at room temperature even without being covered with another cookie. The first version below is your basic plain vanilla. Chocolate and lemon variations follow. Using meringue powder in the filling thickens it and helps it set up quite well when it sits at room temperature (for more on meringue powder, see page 13). In a pinch, you can leave out the meringue powder and try using more confectioners' sugar or less milk for a properly stiff filling, but it simply won't be as stiff or stable. This filling, in all variations, is best made the same day that it will be used as it tends to harden over time, which makes it more difficult to pipe.

10 tablespoons (140 g) unsalted butter, at room temperature

2 tablespoons (1 fluid ounce) milk, at room temperature

1 tablespoon pure vanilla extract

⅛ teaspoon kosher salt

2 teaspoons meringue powder

4 cups (460 g) confectioners' sugar

In the bowl of a stand mixer fitted with the paddle attachment, or a large bowl with a hand mixer, place the butter, milk, and vanilla, and beat on medium speed until combined. Raise the speed to high and beat until creamy. Add the salt, meringue powder, and about 3½ cups of the confectioners' sugar. Mix slowly until the sugar is incorporated. Beat at high speed until uniformly thick. Add up to the remaining ½ cup of the confectioners' sugar, if necessary, to thicken the frosting.

CHOCOLATE VARIATION: In place of the 4 cups (460 g) of confectioners' sugar, use 3½ cups (400 g) of confectioners' sugar plus ¾ cup (60 g) of unsweetened cocoa powder. Begin by adding 3 cups (345 g) of the confectioners' sugar and all the cocoa powder along with the meringue powder. Then, add up to the remaining ½ cup of the confectioners' sugar, if necessary, to thicken the frosting.

LEMON VARIATION: Replace 1 tablespoon of the milk with the juice of 1 lemon, and add finely grated zest of 1 lemon.

Peanut Butter Filling

4 tablespoons (56 g) unsalted butter, chopped

¾ cup (192 g) no-stir smooth peanut butter

½ teaspoon pure vanilla extract

¼ teaspoon kosher salt

1 cup (115 g) confectioners' sugar

1 to 2 tablespoons (½ to 1 fluid ounce) heavy whipping cream

Whenever this peanut butter filling is called for (such as in Do-Si-Dos, page 46, and Ritz Bits Peanut Butter Sandwich Crackers, page 193), natural peanut butter (the type that separates in the jar) can be used in place of the regular no-stir smooth peanut butter called for here. But it won't taste just like the original version of the snack, and it also won't be stable enough to sandwich between two cookies and crackers without sneaking out the sides. This filling is best made the same day that it will be used as it begins to harden over time, which makes it hard to pipe.

In a small, heavy-bottomed saucepan, heat the butter and peanut butter over medium heat, stirring frequently, until just melted. Remove the pan from the heat, add the vanilla, salt, and confectioners' sugar, and stir until well combined. The mixture will be very thick. Add 1 tablespoon of the cream, and stir to thin the filling. Add up to another tablespoon of cream, if necessary, to create a thickly pourable filling. Allow the filling to cool until no longer hot to the touch.

CHAPTER 3

Snack Cakes

The Miniature Cakes You Remember —but Better

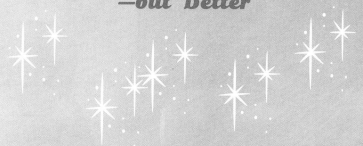

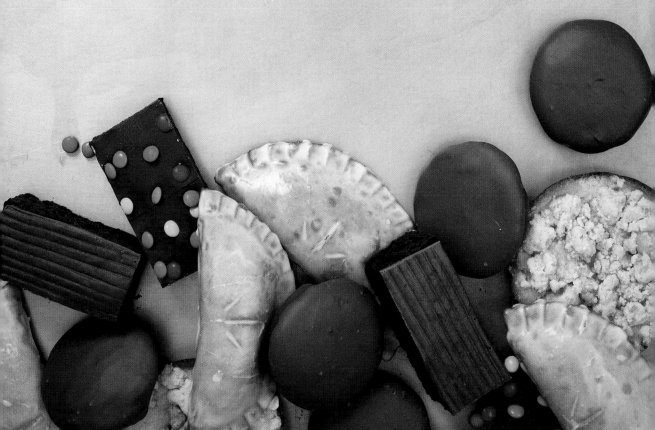

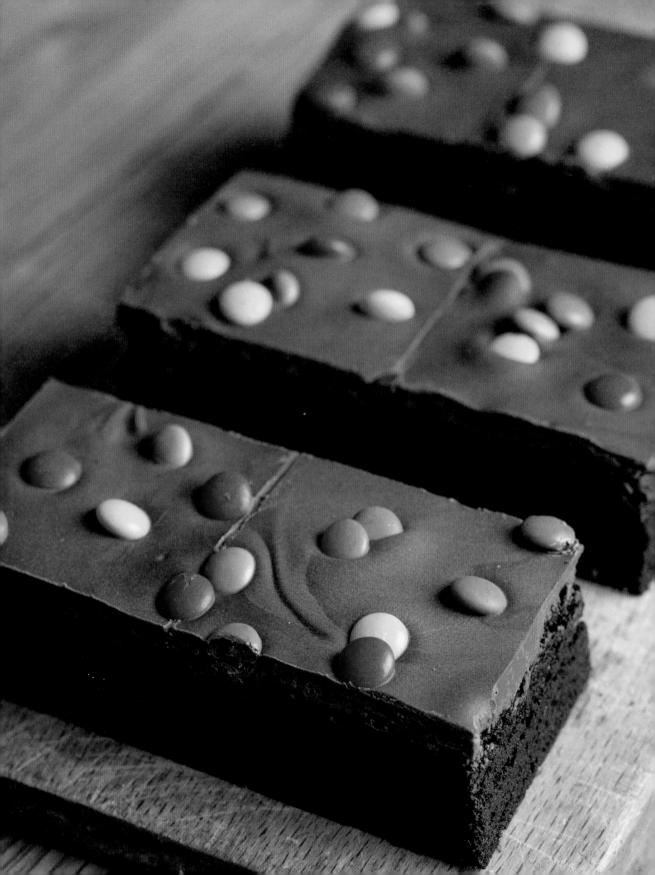

Little Debbie Cosmic Brownies

MAKES 12 BROWNIES

Brownies

1 cup (140 g) all-purpose gluten-free flour (see page 2)

¾ cup (60 g) unsweetened cocoa powder

⅛ teaspoon kosher salt

¾ cup (150 g) granulated sugar

½ cup (109 g) packed light brown sugar

8 tablespoons (112 g) unsalted butter, at room temperature

2 tablespoons (28 g) canola oil

2 teaspoons pure vanilla extract

2 tablespoons (42 g) light corn syrup

2 eggs (100 g, weighed out of shell), at room temperature, beaten

CONTINUED ON PAGE 114

There is indeed something special about Little Debbie brownies. It's not *just* the superfudgy brownie layer and the frosting-like chocolate topping, neither of which ever becomes completely solid even when you put them in the freezer. And it's not *just* the multicolored candy-coated chocolates on top. It's also that seam in the middle that makes the brownies easy to split and share! Although I'm fairly certain I've never actually shared a Little Debbie brownie, knowing that I could do it so easily somehow makes me feel generous. So for true authenticity, be sure not to skip making that seam as your last step.

Prepare the brownies: Preheat your oven to 350°F. Grease and line an 8-inch square pan with two sheets of unbleached parchment paper, crisscrossed in the pan with enough paper to overhang all the edges, and set it aside.

In a large bowl, place the flour, cocoa powder, salt, and granulated sugar, and whisk to combine well. Add the brown sugar and whisk again, working out any lumps. Create a well in the center of the dry ingredients, and add the butter, oil, vanilla, corn syrup, and eggs, mixing to combine after each addition. The batter should be thick and smooth. Scrape it into the prepared baking pan and spread into an even layer with a moist spatula. Place in the center of the preheated oven and bake until just firm to the touch and a toothpick inserted into the center comes out mostly clean, 25 to 28 minutes. Allow to cool completely in the pan.

When the brownies are nearly cool, prepare the topping: Place the chocolate in a medium-size, heatproof bowl, and set it aside. Place the cream in a small, heavy-bottomed saucepan and bring to a simmer over medium-low heat. Add the salt to the cream and stir to combine. Pour the warm cream over the chopped chocolate and allow to

CONTINUED FROM PAGE 113

Topping

8 ounces semisweet chocolate, chopped

2/3 cup (5 1/3 fluid ounces) heavy whipping cream

1/8 teaspoon kosher salt

3 ounces miniature M&Ms candies or multicolored Sixlets, for decorating

sit until the chocolate begins to melt. Stir until the chocolate is melted and smooth. Allow the mixture to cool for about 2 minutes before pouring over the cooled brownies, still in the pan, in an even layer. Scatter the miniature M&Ms (Ms side down, if you're being fastidious) over the chocolate layer, and allow to set at room temperature for about 30 minutes before transferring to the refrigerator. Allow to chill in the refrigerator until firm, about another 30 minutes. Remove from the refrigerator and lift the brownies out of the pan, using the overhanging edges of the sheets of parchment paper in the pan. Place on a cutting board and slice the brownies into twelve equal rectangles. With a butter knife, create a seam widthwise down the center of each brownie.

These can be covered and stored at room temperature for up to 3 days. For longer storage, seal tightly in a freezer-safe wrap or bag, and freeze for up to 2 months. Defrost at room temperature. The chocolate coating may bloom a bit over time, but it won't affect the taste at all.

Little Debbie Oatmeal Creme Pies

MAKES 12 SANDWICH COOKIES

The oatmeal cookies in Little Debbie Oatmeal Creme Pies are the perfect texture for an oatmeal cookie sandwich: not crispy, and not thick and chewy. Instead, they're thin and chewy, but without being fragile, and they give way perfectly to the sweet, lightweight filling inside that sets off the hearty oats just right. The cookies are very soft when they first come out of the oven, so be sure to let them set on the baking sheet as directed. Once they cool, they will reach that perfect Little Debbie-like consistency.

First, prepare the cookies: Preheat your oven to 325°F. Line rimmed baking sheets with unbleached parchment paper and set them aside.

In a large bowl, place the flour, processed oats, baking soda, salt, and granulated sugar, and whisk to combine well. Add the brown sugar and whisk again, working out any lumps. Create a well in the center of the dry ingredients and add the butter, shortening, egg, molasses, vanilla, and cornstarch-dusted raisins, mixing to combine after each addition. The dough should be thick. Divide it into 1½-inch balls. Roll them into smooth balls between your palms and press into disks about ¼ inch thick. Place about 2 inches apart from one another on the prepared baking sheets, and place in the freezer for about 10 minutes, or until firm. Remove from the freezer and place in the center of the preheated oven. Bake until the cookies are lightly golden brown all over and set in the center, 12 to 14 minutes. Allow to cool on the baking sheets for 10 minutes before transferring to a wire rack to cool completely.

While the cookies are cooling, make the Stiff Sandwich Cookie Filling: Follow the directions on page 109, but add more milk by the teaspoonful, beating well after each addition, until the filling is a bit softer but will still hold its shape. Transfer the filling to a pastry bag fitted with a ½-inch plain piping tip and invert half of the cookies. Once the cookies

Cookies

1½ cups (210 g) all-purpose gluten-free flour (see page 2)

1¼ cups (125 g) certified gluten-free old-fashioned rolled oats, processed in a blender or food processor until only a few large pieces remain

¾ teaspoon baking soda

¼ teaspoon kosher salt

¼ cup (50 g) granulated sugar

¾ cup (164 g) packed light brown sugar

5 tablespoons (70 g) unsalted butter, at room temperature

4 tablespoons (48 g) nonhydrogenated vegetable shortening, melted and cooled

1 egg (50 g, weighed out of shell), at room temperature, beaten

CONTINUED ON PAGE 117

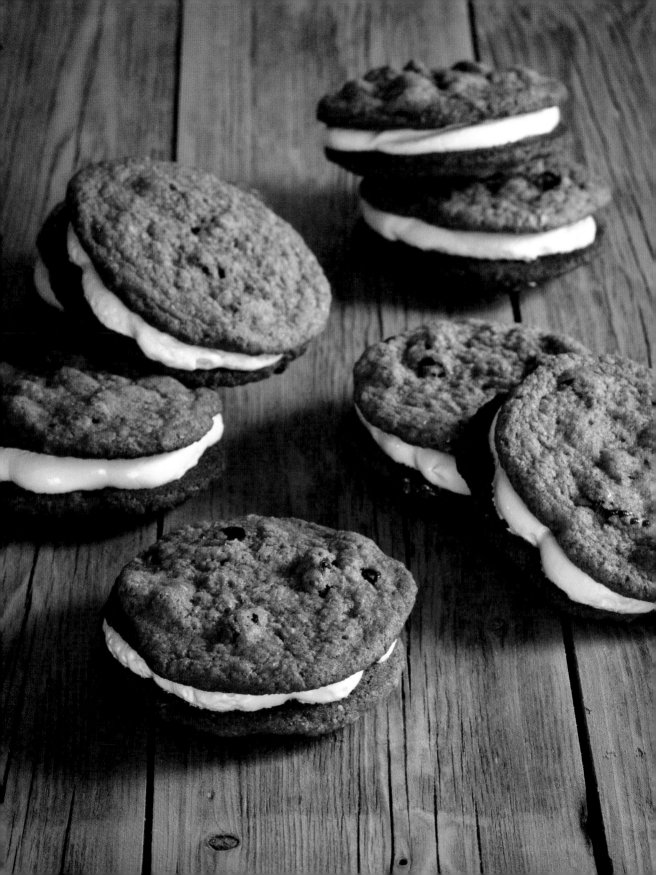

are cool, pipe about 3 tablespoons of filling on the inverted cookies and top with the other cookies to form a sandwich.

The filled snack cakes can be stored in a sealed glass container at room temperature and should maintain their texture for at least 2 days. For longer storage, seal the unfilled cookies tightly in a freezer-safe wrap or bag, and freeze for up to 2 months. Defrost at room temperature and fill as directed.

CONTINUED FROM PAGE 115

2 tablespoons (42 g) unsulfured molasses

1 teaspoon pure vanilla extract

6 ounces raisins, tossed with 1 teaspoon cornstarch

Filling

Stiff Sandwich Cookie Filling (page 109), thinned with another 1 to 2 tablespoons milk

Little Debbie Swiss Rolls

MAKES 6 SNACK CAKES

Cakes

4 eggs (200 g, weighed out of shell), at room temperature, separated

¾ cup (150 g) granulated sugar

6 tablespoons (84 g) unsalted butter, melted and cooled

1 tablespoon warm water

½ cup (70 g) all-purpose gluten-free flour (see page 2)

5 tablespoons (25 g) unsweetened cocoa powder

1 tablespoon (9 g) cornstarch

¼ teaspoon kosher salt

Confectioners' sugar, for rolling

CONTINUED ON PAGE 120

*L*ittle Debbie calls them Swiss Rolls, Hostess calls them Ho-Hos, and Drake's calls them Yodels. I grew up with Yodels and loved eating them chilled, so I could eat them properly: by peeling as much of the chocolate glaze as possible off the rich chocolate cake, all without disturbing the cake. Otherwise, you might be done in just a few minutes without paying this most special of snack cakes the extra attention it's due. I prefer the denser 7-Minute Crème Filling for Snack Cakes for these cakes but the lighter Stabilized Whipped Cream works well, too. There's no need for a special pan here—just a rimmed baking sheet or jelly-roll pan. I have tried using Wilton's special Swiss roll cake pan, with individual baking cavities to make individual rolls that do not need to be sliced into smaller snack cakes, but I found that it was just too easy to overbake the cakes. And even slightly overbaked cakes tend to crack as you try to roll them, so let's avoid that at all costs!

Prepare the cakes: Preheat your oven to 350°F. Line a 13 x 18-inch rimmed baking sheet with unbleached parchment paper and set it aside.

In a large bowl, place the egg yolks, ½ cup (100 g) of the granulated sugar, the butter, and water, and whisk vigorously until pale yellow and smooth. In a separate bowl, place the flour, cocoa powder, cornstarch, and salt, and whisk to combine well. Add the dry ingredients to the egg yolk mixture slowly, while whisking vigorously. The mixture should be thick but smooth. Set it aside.

In the bowl of a stand mixer fitted with the whisk, or a large bowl with a hand mixer, place the egg whites and beat on medium-high speed until soft peaks form. Add the remaining ¼ cup (50 g) of granulated sugar, and continue to beat on medium-high speed until the glossy

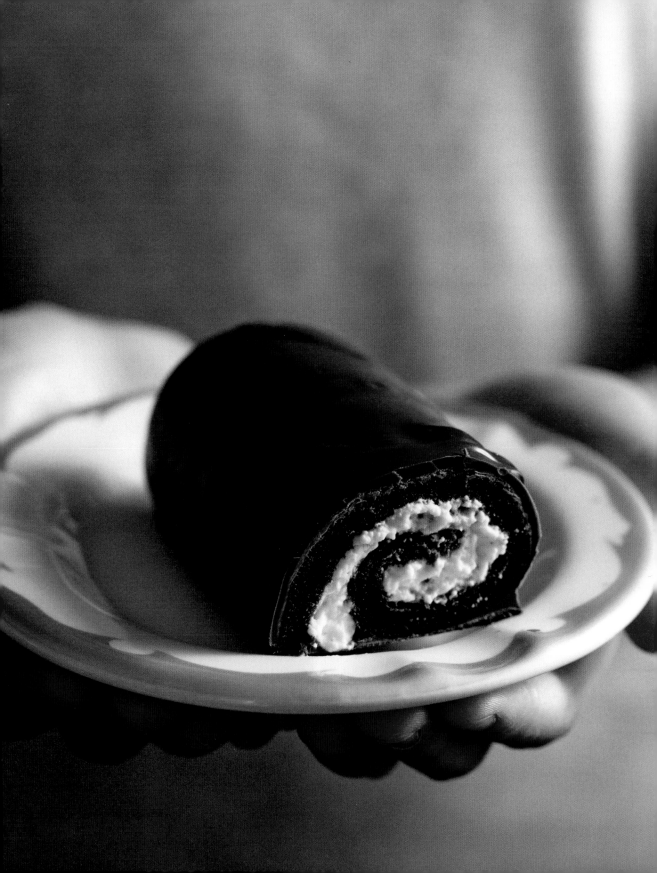

CONTINUED FROM PAGE 118

Filling

7-Minute Crème Filling for Snack Cakes (page 169) or Stabilized Whipped Cream for Snack Cakes (page 170)

Chocolate Glaze

14 ounces semisweet chocolate, chopped

3 tablespoons (42 g) virgin coconut oil

peaks form. Add the egg yolk mixture to the beaten egg whites, and beat until just combined. The batter will be fluffy. Pour it into the prepared baking sheet and spread into an even layer with a bench scraper or offset spatula.

Lay out two tea towels (flat-weave kitchen towels) flat, sprinkle them both generously with confectioners' sugar, and set them aside. Place the baking sheet in the center of the preheated oven and bake for 12 to 14 minutes, or until the cake springs back when pressed gently.

Working quickly with the warm cake, directly out of the oven, invert the baking sheet with the cake on it onto one of the prepared tea towels. Remove the parchment paper from what was the underside of the cake. You now have a bare cake on a sugared tea towel. Using a knife or kitchen shears, cut the cake in half width-wise, creating two smaller and wider halves. Transfer one half to the other confectioners' sugar–dusted towel. Dust the top of each cake with confectioners' sugar and roll it cake away from you, rolling the towel right into the spiral. Repeat with the other cake. Allow both to cool completely, coiled in their towels, on a wire rack.

While the cakes are cooling, prepare the 7-Minute Crème Filling or Stabilized Whipped Cream. Unroll the cakes one at time, remove the tea towel, and spread the filling ¼ inch thick on top of each cake, leaving a ¼-inch border clean all around each cake. Reroll the cakes tightly around the filling (no towels this time) and chill until firm. Once chilled, cut each cake roll by cross-section into three equal pieces, return the snack cakes to the wire rack, and place the rack over a piece of parchment or waxed paper.

Prepare the glaze: In a small, heat-safe bowl, melt the chocolate and coconut oil according to the instructions on page 21. Allow the chocolate to sit at room temperature until it begins to thicken a bit. Pour the glaze over the tops of the filled cakes while still on the wire rack, leaving the two ends exposed. Allow the glaze to set at room temperature.

These snack cakes are best enjoyed within 2 days of being made, but they will keep for up to a month wrapped individually in freezer-safe wrap and frozen. Defrost at room temperature. The chocolate coating may bloom a bit over time, but it won't affect the taste at all.

Little Debbie Zebra Cakes

MAKES 7 CAKES

Some of the other distinctively shaped snack cakes, such as Twinkies (page 129) and Sno Balls (page 137), really must be made in a specialty pan to get the shape just right. But for zebra cakes, all you need for the perfect shape is a six-sided cookie cutter that's about 3 inches across (see Resources, page 294). If you don't have one of those lying around, it's not too difficult to freestyle that shape with a knife. Just try to make at least one cake shaped just right, to guarantee that everyone knows exactly what you've made when you start icing and frosting and drizzling on the zebra stripes.

First, make the cake: Preheat your oven to 325°F. Grease and line a 9 x 12-inch baking pan with unbleached parchment paper and set it aside.

In the bowl of a stand mixer fitted with the paddle attachment, or a large bowl with a hand mixer, place the butter and beat on medium-high speed until light and fluffy. Add the confectioners' sugar, egg, vanilla, and sour cream, mixing to combine well after each addition. In a small bowl, place the cake flour, baking soda, and salt and whisk to combine well. Add the dry ingredients and the milk alternately to the wet mixture, beginning and ending with the dry ingredients, and beating after each addition until just combined. It should be a thickly pourable batter. Pour the batter into the prepared pan, and shake and spread into an even layer.

Place in the center of the preheated oven and bake until the cake springs back when pressed gently in the center, about 25 minutes. Remove the cake from the oven and allow to cool in the pan for 15 minutes before transferring to a wire rack to cool completely. Meanwhile, prepare the 7-Minute Crème Filling or Stabilized Whipped Cream.

Place the cooled cake in the freezer until firm, about 10 minutes. This will make it much easier to cut out shapes. Once the cake is firm,

Cake

8 tablespoons (112 g) unsalted butter, at room temperature

1¾ cups (200 g) confectioners' sugar

1 egg (50 g, weighed out of shell), at room temperature, beaten

1 teaspoons pure vanilla extract

½ cup (120 g) sour cream, at room temperature

1 cup (140 g) gluten-free cake flour (see page 2)

½ teaspoon baking soda

¼ teaspoon kosher salt

½ cup (4 fluid ounces) milk, at room temperature

CONTINUED ON PAGE 122

CONTINUED FROM PAGE 121

Filling

7-Minute Crème Filling for Snack Cakes (page 169) or Stabilized Whipped Cream for Snack Cakes (page 170)

White Icing

6 cups (690 g) confectioners' sugar

½ cup (4 fluid ounces) water

2 tablespoons (42 g) light corn syrup

Fudge Stripes

2 ounces semisweet chocolate, chopped

1 teaspoon (5 g) virgin coconut oil

remove it from the freezer and cut out six-sided geometric shapes, each about 3 inches wide, with an appropriate cookie cutter (see Resources, page 294) or a sharp knife. Cut each cake in half horizontally with a sharp knife, spread about 3 tablespoons of the filling on one half, and top with the other half. Set the filled cakes on a wire rack over a rimmed baking sheet or piece of parchment or waxed paper, and set them aside.

Prepare the white icing: Combine all the icing ingredients in a small saucepan, whisk well, and attach a candy thermometer to the side of the pan. Cook over low heat until the mixture reaches 100°F. Pour the warm icing immediately over the shaped and filled cakes. Allow to set at room temperature (or in the refrigerator). If the icing is too translucent on the cakes, warm it again (keeping the temperature below 100°F) and pour another layer over each cake, then allow to set, about 30 minutes.

Prepare the fudge stripes: In a small, heat-safe bowl, melt the chocolate together with the coconut oil as described on page 25. Transfer the melted chocolate to a pastry bag fitted with a very small (a #2 works well) tip, and pipe zebra stripes on the set white icing on each cake. Allow to finish setting at room temperature.

These snack cakes are best enjoyed the day they are finished. The six-sided cut cakes can be made ahead of time, wrapped tightly in freezer-safe wrap, and frozen for up to 2 months. Defrost at room temperature before filling, icing, and decorating as directed.

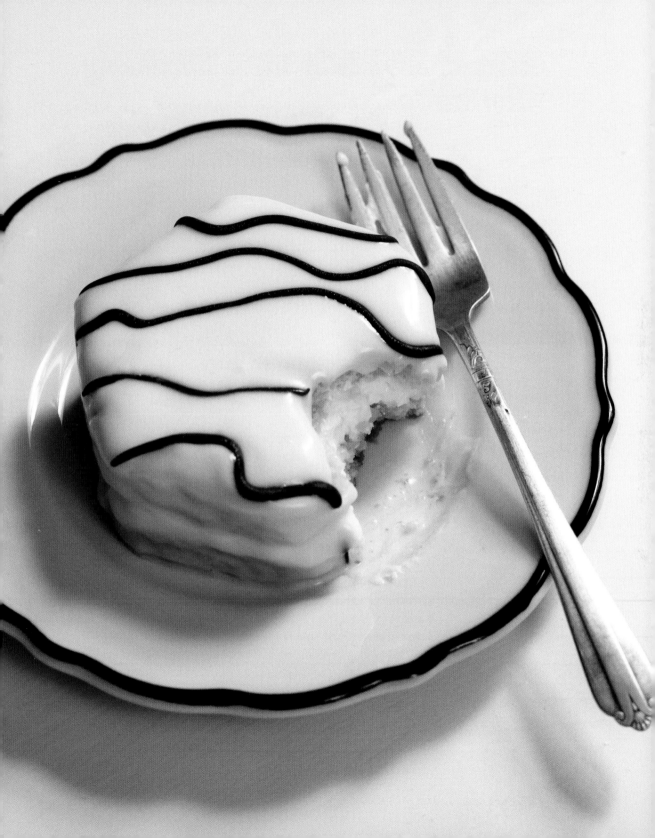

Entenmann's Little Bites Blueberry Muffins

MAKES ABOUT 35 MINI MUFFINS

1 cup plus 2 tablespoons (158 g) all-purpose gluten-free flour (see page 2)

¼ cup (36 g) cornstarch

1 teaspoon baking powder

⅛ teaspoon baking soda

½ teaspoon kosher salt

6 tablespoons (75 g) granulated sugar

2 tablespoons (28 g) unsalted butter, at room temperature

2 tablespoons (28 g) canola oil

½ cup (4 fluid ounces) milk, at room temperature

2 eggs (100 g), at room temperature, beaten

⅔ cup (80 g) whole fresh blueberries, tossed with 1 teaspoon cornstarch

*A*s many times as I have made blueberry muffins for my children, they still begged for Little Bites, since apparently *allllll* their friends at the school lunch table had them. I tried to explain to them that Little Bites were just miniature versions of the blueberry muffins I had already been making. But when I got to work on this copycat recipe, I remembered how different they really were. Light and airy but still tender and lightly sweet, Little Bites are worthy of all the hype among the grade school set.

Preheat your oven to 350°F. Grease very well the bottom and halfway up the sides of twenty-four miniature muffin cups. Do not grease the very top of the sides of the muffin wells. The ungreased area coaxes the muffins into rising into a dome, instead of flattening on top.

In a large bowl, place the flour, cornstarch, baking powder, baking soda, salt, and sugar, and whisk to combine well. Create a well in the center of the dry ingredients, and add the butter, oil, milk, and eggs, mixing to combine after each addition. The batter should be thick and fluffy. Add the cornstarch-dusted blueberries, folding them gently into the batter until they are evenly distributed throughout the dough, and taking care not to break the berries. Fill the prepared muffin cups all the way full and, using wet fingers, flatten the tops.

Place in the center of the preheated oven and bake until the center of each muffin bounces back when pressed gently, about 15 minutes. Remove from the oven and allow to cool in the muffin tin for 10 minutes before transferring to a wire rack to cool completely.

These muffins will keep in a sealed plastic or glass container at room temperature for up to 3 days. For longer storage, seal them tightly in a freezer-safe wrap or bag, and freeze for up to 2 months. Defrost at room temperature.

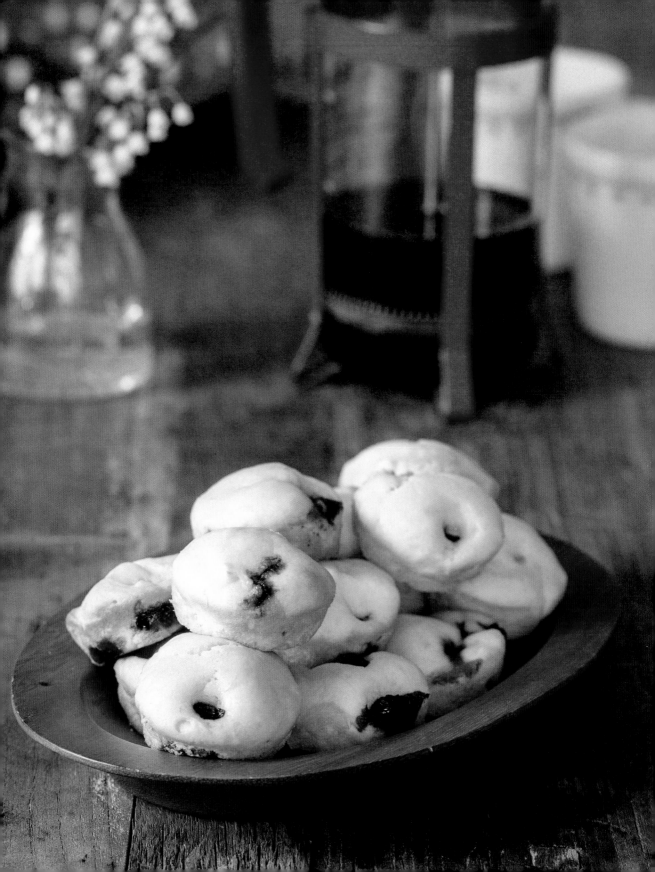

Entenmann's Little Bites Chocolate Chip Muffins

MAKES ABOUT 35 MINI MUFFINS

1 cup plus 2 tablespoons
(158 g) all-purpose
gluten-free flour (see
page 2)

¼ cup (36 g) cornstarch

1 teaspoon baking powder

⅛ teaspoon baking soda

½ teaspoon kosher salt

¼ cup (50 g) granulated
sugar

¼ cup (55 g) packed
light brown sugar

2 tablespoons (28 g)
unsalted butter, at room
temperature

2 tablespoons (28 g)
canola oil

½ cup (4 fluid ounces)
milk

2 eggs (100 g, weighed
out of shell), at room
temperature, beaten

3 ounces miniature
semisweet chocolate
chips, tossed with
1 teaspoon cornstarch

These chocolate chip Little Bites feel more like a splurge, while the blueberry mini muffins (page 124) seem more like an everyday treat. Anything with chocolate chips in it is cause for celebration in my house, and it doesn't hurt that the moist cake in these chocolate chip miniature muffins is a bit sweeter than the cake in the blueberry ones.

Preheat your oven to 350°F. Grease very well the bottom and halfway up the sides of twenty-four miniature muffin cups. Do not grease the very top of the sides of the muffin wells. The ungreased area coaxes the muffins into rising into a dome, instead of flattening on top.

In a large bowl, place the flour, cornstarch, baking powder, baking soda, salt, and granulated sugar, and whisk to combine well. Add the brown sugar and whisk again, working out any lumps. Create a well in the center of the dry ingredients, and add the butter, oil, milk, and eggs, mixing to combine after each addition. The batter should be thick and fluffy. Add the cornstarch-dusted miniature chips, folding them gently into the batter until they are evenly distributed throughout the dough. Fill the prepared muffin cups all the way full and, using wet fingers, flatten the tops.

Place in the center of the preheated oven and bake until center of each muffin bounces back when pressed gently, about 15 minutes. Remove from the oven and allow to cool in the muffin tin for 10 minutes before transferring to a wire rack to cool completely.

These muffins will keep in a sealed plastic or glass container at room temperature for up to 3 days. For longer storage, seal them tightly in a freezer-safe wrap or bag, and freeze for up to 2 months. Defrost at room temperature.

Entenmann's Little Bites Brownies

MAKES ABOUT 25 MINI MUFFINS

*N*o one is pretending that these sweet little miniature brownies are anything other than an indulgence, but they're such a *small* indulgence that it hardly seems like anything to feel guilty about. They're not the dense, fudgy brownies you expect from, say, Little Debbie Cosmic Brownies (page 113). Instead, they're like a cross between chocolate cake and a brownie, with all the best characteristics of each.

Preheat your oven to 325°F. Grease very well the bottom of and halfway up the sides of twenty-four miniature muffin cups. Do not grease the very top of the sides of the muffin wells. The ungreased area coaxes the brownies into rising into a dome, instead of flattening on top.

In a large bowl, place the flour, cocoa powder, salt, and baking soda, and whisk to combine well. Create a well in the center of the dry ingredients, and place the butter, sour cream, granulated sugar, brown sugar, eggs, and vanilla, mixing to combine well after each addition. The batter will be thick and glossy. Divide the batter evenly among the prepared muffin cups. Shake the muffin tin back and forth vigorously until the batter in each cup is smooth and even on top.

Place the tin in the center of the preheated oven and bake until the brownies are puffed and round, and a toothpick inserted into the center comes out clean, about 12 minutes. Remove from the oven and allow to cool in the muffin tin for 10 minutes before transferring to a wire rack to cool completely.

These brownies will keep in a sealed plastic or glass container at room temperature for up to 3 days. For longer storage, seal them tightly in a freezer-safe wrap or bag, and freeze for up to 2 months. Defrost at room temperature.

---

1 cup (140 g) all-purpose gluten-free flour (see page 2)

½ cup (40 g) unsweetened cocoa powder

¼ teaspoon kosher salt

¼ teaspoon baking soda

6 tablespoons (84 g) unsalted butter, melted and cooled

2 tablespoons (30 g) sour cream, at room temperature

½ cup (100 g) granulated sugar

½ cup (109 g) packed light brown sugar

2 eggs (100 g, weighed out of shell), at room temperature, beaten

1 teaspoon pure vanilla extract

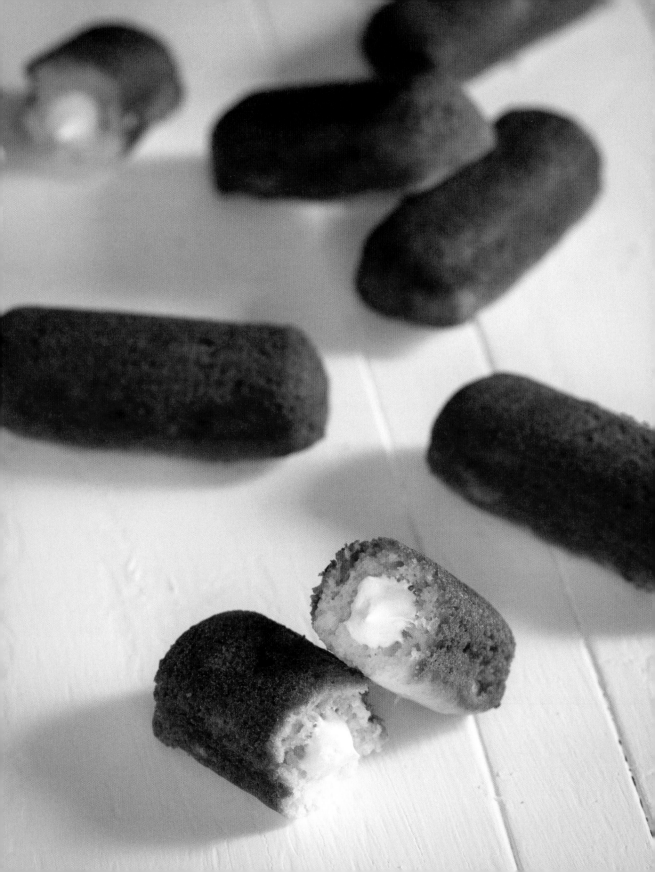

Hostess Twinkies

MAKES 12 CAKES

The chiffon-style cake batter in these Twinkie-style snack cakes is very good at rising without much of a dome on top, creating a very authentic-looking snack cake. The moist and sweet yellow cakes are light and airy, just like the original, due in part to the use of gluten-free cake flour. If you are aiming for the perfect authentic shape, Hostess itself makes a "Twinkie" pan. I haven't tried it myself, but I bet it makes just the best Twinkies ever. Other options are Wilton's twelve-cavity Delectovals Cake Pan and Norpro's Cream Canoe Pan. If you can live without the Twinkie shape, they taste just as delicious when you make them as cupcakes. As with many of the other Hostess-style filled snack cakes, I have a slight preference for the lighter Stabilized Whipped Cream for Snack Cakes, but either filling will do just fine.

Prepare the cakes: Preheat your oven to 350°F. Grease twelve single-serving wells of an appropriate canoe-shaped snack cake pan (or a standard twelve-cup muffin tin) and set it aside.

In a large bowl, place the cake flour, baking powder, baking soda, salt, and sugar, and whisk to combine well. Create a well in the center of the dry ingredients, and add the shortening, butter, and milk, whisking vigorously to combine well after each addition. In the bowl of a stand mixer fitted with the whisk attachment, or a large bowl with a hand mixer, whip the egg whites until stiff (but not dry) peaks form. Add about half of the whipped egg whites to the batter and whisk to combine well. Add the remaining egg whites and carefully fold into the batter until no white streaks remain.

Divide the batter evenly among the prepared wells of the pan. Place the pan in the center of the preheated oven and bake until a toothpick inserted into the center of a cake comes out clean, about 16 minutes.

Cakes

1½ cups (210 g) gluten-free cake flour (see page 2)

1 teaspoon baking powder

½ teaspoon baking soda

½ teaspoon kosher salt

1 cup (200 g) granulated sugar

2 tablespoons (24 g) nonhydrogenated vegetable shortening, melted and cooled

2 tablespoons (28 g) unsalted butter, melted and cooled

⅔ cup (5⅓ fluid ounces) milk, at room temperature

4 egg whites (100 g), at room temperature

Filling

Stabilized Whipped Cream for Snack Cakes (page 170) or 7-Minute Crème Filling for Snack Cakes (page 169)

Allow to cool in the pan for 10 minutes before inverting the cakes (flat-side down) and transferring to a wire rack to cool completely.

Prepare the Stabilized Whipped Cream or 7-Minute Crème Filling. Once the cakes are cool, transfer them to a flat surface lined with parchment or waxed paper. Using a toothpick or wooden skewer, poke three evenly spaced holes in the bottom of each cake, wiggling the skewer around a bit to create some space inside the cakes. Transfer the filling to a pastry bag fitted with a Bismarck tip, and pipe filling into each of the three holes in each snack cake until the holes are filled and a bit of filling peaks out of each hole.

These snack cakes are best enjoyed within 2 days of being filled, but they will keep for up to a month wrapped individually in freezer-safe wrap and frozen. Defrost at room temperature.

Hostess Chocolate Cupcakes

MAKES 18 CUPCAKES

*E*verybody knows that rich Hostess chocolate cupcakes, crème-filled, topped with chocolate and a perfect swirl of white icing, are moist and delicious. Everybody knows (don't they?) that they are not baked in cupcake liners. They must have smooth sides, not the ridges created by liners. And unlike Drake's Ring Dings (page 155), they are dense chocolate cakes, not devil's food cake—made here with *real* chocolate, not cocoa powder. You can't very well maintain your dignity if you put out a cookbook filled with snack cakes and not have it include the perfect version of these iconic gems. Lucky for me (and my dignity), these cupcakes have just the right everything: taste, texture, and appearance. They've got it all. Either suggested filling works, but I prefer the lighter Stabilized Whipped Cream for Snack Cakes for the most authentic Hostess-style chocolate cupcake.

Prepare the cupcakes: Preheat your oven to 350°F. Grease the wells of a standard twelve-cup muffin tin well and set it aside.

In a medium-size, heat-safe bowl, place the chocolate and butter and melt as instructed on page 21. To the bowl of melted chocolate and butter, add the sugar, sour cream, egg, and vanilla, beating well after each addition. In a large bowl, place the flour, cocoa powder, baking powder, baking soda, and salt, and whisk to combine well. Create a well in the center of the dry ingredients, add the wet ingredients, and mix to combine. The batter will be thick.

Fill the prepared muffin cups two-thirds full and shake the batter into an even layer in each well. Place the pan in the center of the preheated oven and bake for about 18 minutes, or until the cupcakes are just firm to the touch. Allow the cupcakes the cool in the muffin tin for 10 minutes

Cupcakes

4½ ounces dark chocolate, chopped

6 tablespoons (84 g) unsalted butter, chopped

1 cup (200 g) granulated sugar

⅔ cup (160 g) sour cream, at room temperature

2 eggs (100 g, weighed out of shell), at room temperature, beaten

1 tablespoon pure vanilla extract

1½ cups (210 g) all-purpose gluten-free flour (see page 2)

¼ cup (20 g) unsweetened cocoa powder

½ teaspoon baking powder

½ teaspoon baking soda

¼ teaspoon kosher salt

CONTINUED ON PAGE 132

CONTINUED FROM PAGE 131

Filling

Stabilized Whipped Cream for Snack Cakes (page 170) or 7-Minute Crème Filling for Snack Cakes (page 169)

Glaze

10 ounces semisweet chocolate, chopped

4 tablespoons (56 g) virgin coconut oil

Swirl

Royal Icing (page 172)

---

before transferring to a wire rack to cool completely. Repeat with the remaining batter.

Prepare the Stabilized Whipped Cream or 7-Minute Crème Filling. Once the cakes have cooled, create a well in the center of the top of each cake with a ¾-inch round cookie cutter, cutting off the bottom with a knife (reserve the removed cake pieces). Transfer the filling to a pastry bag fitted with a ¼-inch plain piping tip and pipe about 1½ tablespoons of prepared filling into the open well in each cake. Cover the filling in each cake with a previously removed cake piece and press down to secure. Place the cakes back on the wire rack over a piece of parchment or waxed paper.

Prepare the glaze: Place the chocolate and coconut oil in a medium-size heat-safe bowl and melt according to the instructions on page 21. Dip the top of each cooled and filled cupcake carefully into the glaze, bob it up and down a few times to ensure that the entire top of each cake is covered in glaze, and invert back onto the wire rack. Allow the glaze to set at room temperature.

Once the chocolate glaze is set, add the swirl: Place the royal icing in a pastry bag with very small (#1 or #2) piping tip, and pipe a swirl across the top of the chocolate glaze. Allow to set once again at room temperature.

These snack cakes are best enjoyed within 2 days of being glazed, but they will keep for up to a month wrapped individually in freezer-safe wrap and frozen. Defrost at room temperature. The chocolate glaze may bloom a bit over time, but it won't affect the taste at all.

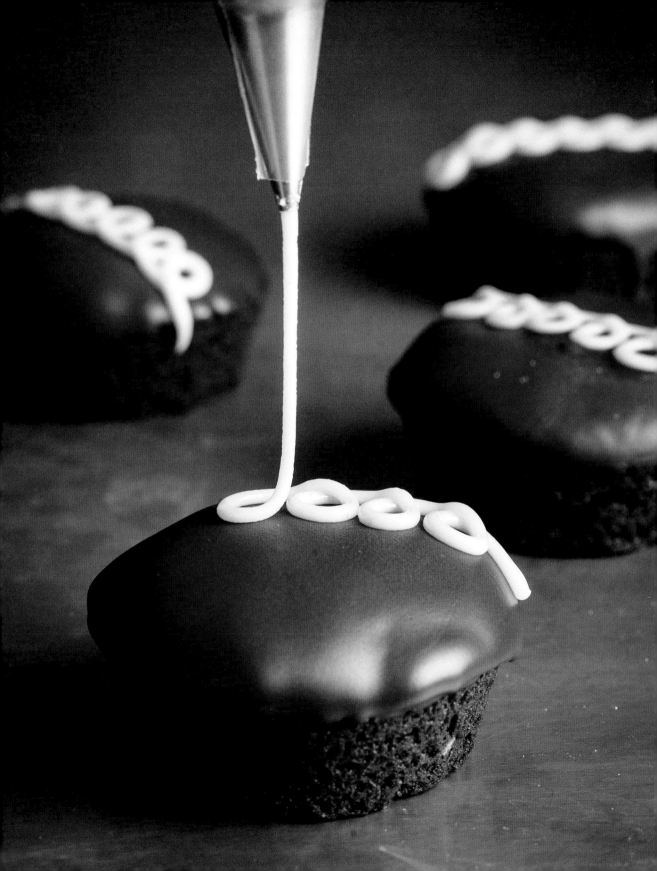

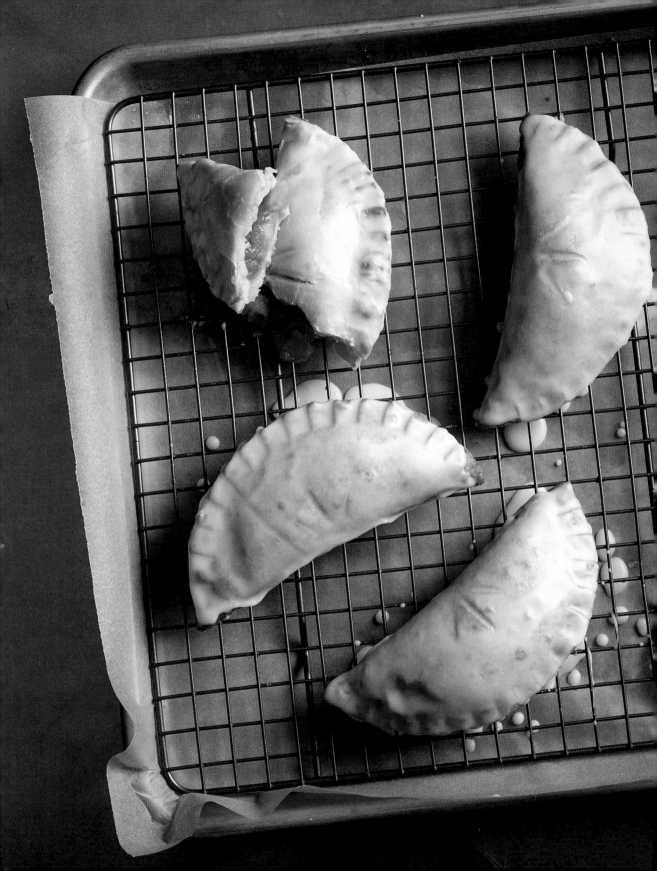

Hostess Apple Fruit Pies

MAKES 10 PIES

*A*pparently, at some point in the last few years, Hostess changed the formulation for its apple fruit pies. I have absolutely no earthly idea why anyone would ever mess with perfection, but they did. These apple fruit pies are in the style of the old-school version. (PS: I think all Hostess did was to stop piling all the filling toward the center as it used to do.) You can make these all in a day, or you can make the filling up to three days ahead of time and store it in a sealed container in the refrigerator. Simply bring it to room temperature before using it to fill the pies.

NOTE: A cake cutter or hand pie cutter will come in handy here to create the pie shapes (see Resources, page 294).

First, prepare the filling ahead so it has time to cool: In a medium, heavy-bottomed saucepan, place all the filling ingredients and cook over medium heat, stirring occasionally, until the apples are soft and the mixture has thickened, about 6 minutes. Remove from the heat and allow to cool to room temperature.

Prepare the crust: In a large bowl, place the flour, cornstarch, salt, and sugar, and whisk to combine well. Create a well in the center of the dry ingredients and add the butter, egg, vanilla, and 2 fluid ounces of the milk, mixing to combine after each addition. Knead the dough with your hands, adding more milk by the half-teaspoonful as necessary to bring the dough together. It should be thick but smooth.

Transfer the dough to a lightly floured surface and sprinkle very lightly with more flour. Roll out into a rectangle about ¼ inch thick. Cut out rounds 6 inches in diameter with a cake cutter or hand pie cutter.

With wet fingers or a wet pastry brush, moisten the border of one crust, and place about ⅓ cup filling off center, concentrating the filling toward the center of the round rather than an even layer all the way across the crust. Fold the crust in half, enclosing the filling, and cinch

Filling

3 firm apples (Empire or Granny Smith work especially well), peeled, cored, and diced

2 tablespoons (18 g) cornstarch

½ cup (109 g) packed light brown sugar

1 teaspoon kosher salt

1 tablespoon (½ fluid ounce) lukewarm water

Crust

2¼ cups (315 g) all-purpose gluten-free flour (see page 2), plus more for sprinkling

¼ cup (36 g) cornstarch

¼ teaspoon kosher salt

¾ cup (150 g) granulated sugar

8 tablespoons (112 g) unsalted butter, at room temperature

CONTINUED ON PAGE 136

CONTINUED FROM PAGE 135

1 egg (50 g, weighed out of shell), at room temperature, beaten

1 teaspoon pure vanilla extract

4 to 6 tablespoons (2 to 3 fluid ounces) milk, at room temperature

Oil, for frying

Glaze

1 cup (115 g) confectioners' sugar

1 teaspoon meringue powder

3 to 5 teaspoons warm water

the edges closed securely. Slash the top of the pie with a sharp knife in three short strokes. Repeat with the remaining filling and crusts.

Place a wire rack above paper towels on a baking sheet and set it aside. Place 2 inches of oil in a heavy-bottomed saucepan or deep fryer. Clip a candy/deep-fry thermometer to the side of the saucepan, and bring the oil to 350°F. Place the pies in the hot oil in small batches, taking care not to crowd them at all. Allow to fry until lightly golden brown all over, about 3 minutes per side. Remove the pies from the oil, and place on the prepared wire rack.

Once the pies are cool, prepare the glaze: In a small bowl, place the confectioners' sugar, meringue powder, and 3 teaspoons of the water and mix to combine well. It should form a thick paste. Add more water by the half-teaspoonful to thin the glaze until it falls off the spoon in a thin ribbon. With the cooled pies still on the wire rack, pour the glaze lightly over them and spread it into an even layer. Allow the glaze to set into a thin shell.

Once they are finished, these apple pies are best enjoyed the day they are made or the following day. I have successfully wrapped them tightly in plastic wrap and sent them in my children's lunchboxes the day after they were made and heard absolutely no complaints. Quite the contrary!

Hostess Sno Balls

MAKES 12 CAKES

*L*ike other snack cakes, homemade Sno Balls can be baked in specialty cake pans from such companies as Wilton (called a 12-Cavity Orb Cake Pan) or Fat Daddio (a Sno Cake Pan or Perfect Pan for Snow Balls, depending upon the source of the product), or in a standard twelve-cup muffin tin, in which case they won't be dome shaped unless you are in a carving mood. Whatever the shape, they'll taste just the same as you remember: a moist and rich chocolate devil's food–style cake, filled with a soft crème, then covered in a layer of marshmallow and topped generously with lightly sweetened coconut flakes. In place of the coconut topping in the recipe, you could simply use packaged sweetened shredded coconut, but I find that it just doesn't taste like coconut. And as they do with the packaged cakes, you can always add some powdered food coloring to the toasted coconut chips when you pulse them in a food processor. For the filling, I prefer the lighter Stabilized Whipped Cream for Snack Cakes, but the choice is yours.

Prepare the cakes: Preheat your oven to 350°F. Grease twelve single-serving wells of an appropriate dome-shaped snack cake pan (or a standard twelve-cup muffin tin) and set it aside.

In the bowl of a stand mixer fitted with the paddle attachment, or a large bowl with a hand mixer, place the butter and beat on medium-high speed until light and fluffy. Add the sugar, eggs, sour cream, and vanilla, beating to combine after each addition. In a small bowl, place the flour, cocoa powder, baking soda, and salt, and whisk to combine well. Add the dry ingredients and water to the bowl of wet ingredients alternately, beginning and ending with the dry ingredients and mixing to combine

Cakes

8 tablespoons (112 g) unsalted butter, at room temperature

1½ cups (327 g) packed light brown sugar

2 eggs (100 g, weighed out of shell), at room temperature

½ cup (120 g) sour cream, at room temperature

1 teaspoon pure vanilla extract

2 cups (280 g) all-purpose gluten-free flour (see page 2)

¾ cup (60 g) unsweetened cocoa powder

1¼ teaspoons baking soda

½ teaspoon kosher salt

1⅓ cups (10⅔ fluid ounces) warm water

CONTINUED ON PAGE 138

CONTINUED FROM PAGE 137

Filling

Stabilized Whipped Cream for Snack Cakes (page 170) or 7-Minute Crème Filling for Snack Cakes (page 169)

Coconut Topping

1½ cups (120 g) coconut flakes

¼ cup (50 g) granulated sugar

2 tablespoons (1 fluid ounce) water

Marshmallow Topping

¾ tablespoon (5 g) unflavored powdered gelatin

½ cup (4 fluid ounces) cool water

1 cup (200 g) granulated sugar

⅛ teaspoon cream of tartar

½ teaspoon pure vanilla extract

⅛ teaspoon kosher salt

well after each addition. Pour the batter into the prepared pan, filling the wells two-thirds full.

Place the pans, one at a time, in the center of the preheated oven and bake until a toothpick inserted into the center of a cake comes out mostly clean, 13 to 15 minutes. Allow to cool in the pan for about 10 minutes before slicing off the rounded top of each cake to make a flat top and placing on a wire rack, cut-side down, to cool completely.

Prepare the Stabilized Whipped Cream or 7-Minute Crème Filling and set it aside.

Prepare the coconut topping: Reduce the oven temperature to 275°F. Line a large rimmed baking sheet with unbleached parchment paper, place the coconut flakes on the baking sheet and set aside. In a small, heavy-bottomed saucepan, place the sugar and water and mix to combine well. Cook over medium heat until the sugar is dissolved, about 2 minutes. Pour the sugar syrup over the coconut flakes on the baking sheet, and toss to combine. Spread out the coconut into an even layer on the baking sheet, and place in the center of the preheated oven. Bake until the coconut is fragrant and beginning to brown on the edges, about 7 minutes. Remove from the oven and allow to cool slightly before pulsing in the food processor until the chips are the size of coarse bread crumbs.

Once the cakes have cooled, create a well in the center of the cut side of each cake with a ¾-inch round cookie cutter, cutting off the bottom with a knife (reserve the removed cake pieces). Transfer the filling to a pastry bag fitted with a ¼-inch plain piping tip and pipe about 1½ tablespoons of the prepared filling into the open well in each cake. Cover the filling in each cake with a previously removed cake piece. Invert the cakes and place them back on the wire rack, placed over a piece of parchment or waxed paper.

Prepare the marshmallow topping: Bloom the gelatin in 2 fluid ounces of the cool water by placing both in the bowl of a stand mixer fitted with the whisk attachment, or a large bowl with a hand mixer, and mixing them together. Allow to sit until the gelatin swells. In a small, heavy-bottomed saucepan, clip a candy thermometer to the side, place the remaining 2 ounces of cool water, and the sugar and cream of tartar, and cook until the mixture reaches 240°F. Pour the hot mixture down the side of the mixer bowl with the bloomed gelatin, add the vanilla and salt, whisk together with a separate, handheld whisk, and allow to cool

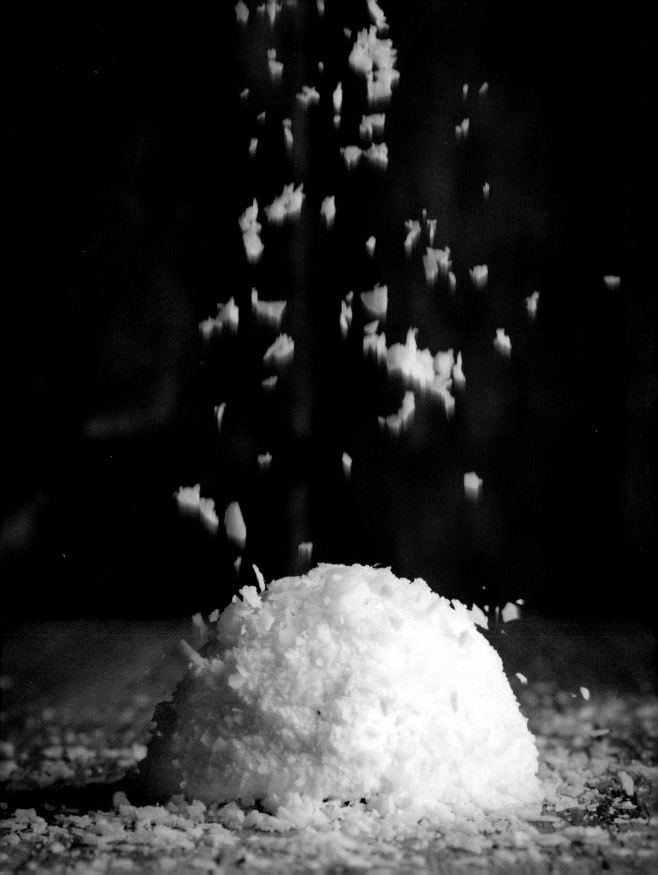

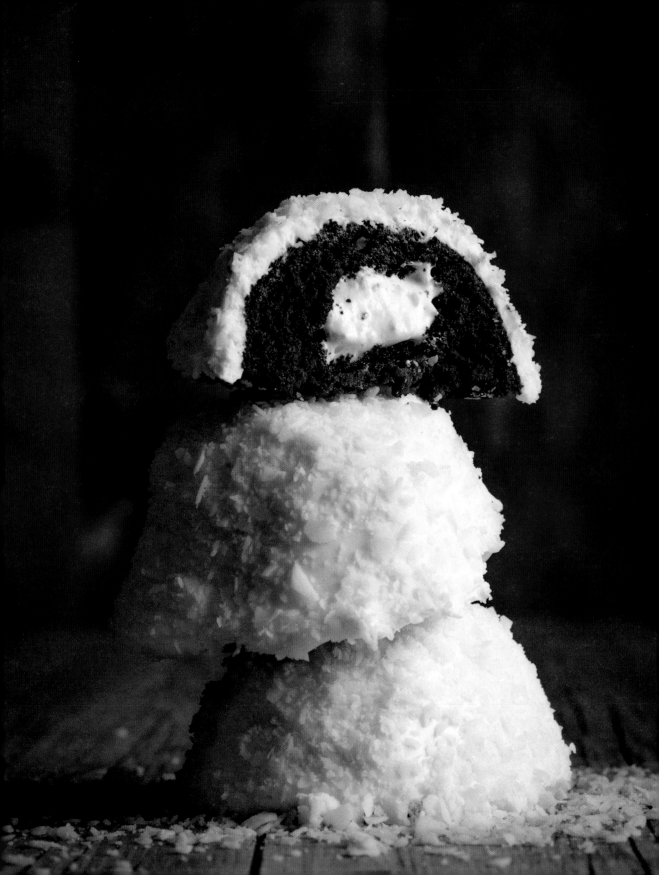

briefly until no longer hot to the touch. Whisk on medium speed until thick, white, and glossy. The marshmallow mixture will triple in size. It is ready when it pours off the beaters slowly. Pour the marshmallow topping thickly over the cooled cakes right away, spreading all over the top of the round cakes. Top the marshmallow on each cake immediately with the coconut topping and press down gently to make sure the coconut adheres. Allow to set at room temperature.

As assembled, these cakes are best enjoyed the day they are made. However, the unfilled cakes themselves may be frozen in a single layer on a baking sheet, then sealed tightly in a freezer-safe wrap or bag, and frozen for up to 2 months. Defrost at room temperature, and then fill and decorate as directed.

Tastykake Butterscotch Krimpets

MAKES 9 CAKES

Butterscotch Sauce

4 tablespoons (56 g) unsalted butter, chopped

½ cup (109 g) packed light brown sugar

¾ cup (150 g) granulated sugar

¾ cup (6 fluid ounces) heavy whipping cream

Pure vanilla extract

Coarse salt

Cakes

2 cups (280 g) all-purpose gluten-free flour (see page 2)

¾ teaspoon baking powder

¼ teaspoon baking soda

½ teaspoon kosher salt

1 cup (200 g) granulated sugar

8 tablespoons (112 g) unsalted butter, at room temperature

CONTINUED ON PAGE 144

I'd like to begin by thanking my husband, who was born and bred in Philadelphia. Growing up, I had never even heard of Krimpets, butterscotch or otherwise. Clearly, I lived a sadly sheltered life. My husband showed me what I'd been missing: moist and rich vanilla- and butterscotch-flavored snack cakes that are "crimped" on the sides into something of a zigzag pattern. The icing is smooth and loaded with a deep, satisfying butterscotch flavor. When you're making your own Krimpets, be sure to prepare the butterscotch sauce first so it has a chance to cool before you add it to the icing. It may seem like a fair amount of work—but it's really quite simple and so worth it.

Prepare the butterscotch sauce: In a medium-size, heavy-bottomed saucepan, place the chopped butter. Place the remaining ingredients in individual small bowls alongside the stovetop, for easy access. Melt the butter over medium-low heat. Add the brown sugar, and stir until the mixture is wet and grainy. Add the granulated sugar, and continue to cook over medium-low heat, stirring occasionally, until the mixture is smooth, about 3 minutes. Add the cream and switch to a using whisk (a flat one is ideal for getting into all the edges of the pan, but a balloon whisk will do just fine). Lower the heat to low, and whisk constantly until the mixture is smooth, about 1 minute. Once the mixture is smooth, bring it to a simmer and continue to cook, whisking occasionally, for about another 5 minutes, or until it is slightly reduced and coats the back of a spoon. Remove from the heat, and add the vanilla and coarse salt to taste. Set the sauce aside to cool.

Prepare the cakes: Preheat your oven to 325°F. Grease a 9 x 12-inch rectangular pan. In a large bowl, place the flour, baking powder, baking soda, salt, and granulated sugar, and whisk to combine well. Create a well in the center of the dry ingredients, and add the butter, milk, egg

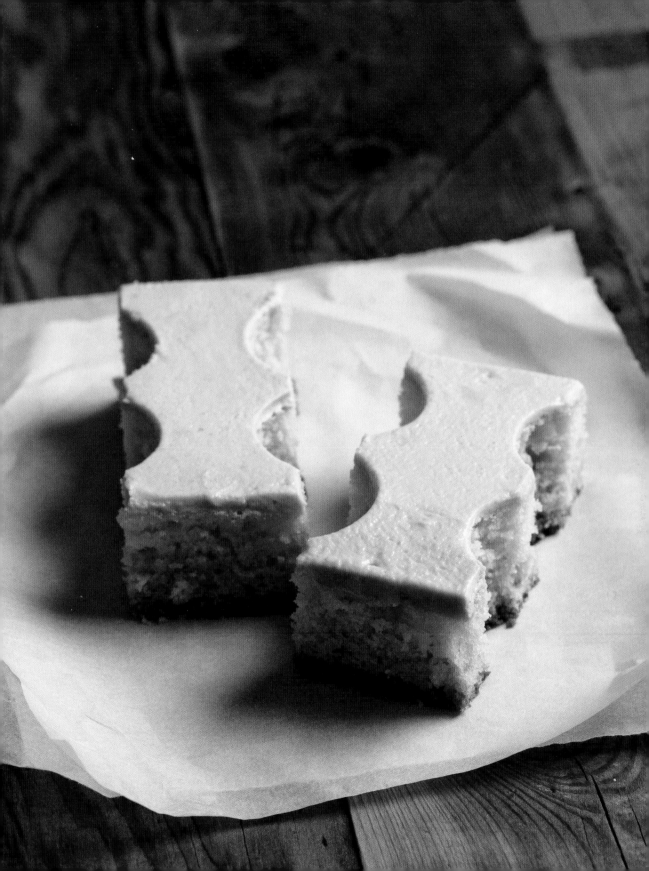

CONTINUED FROM PAGE 142

1 cup (8 fluid ounces) milk, at room temperature

2 egg yolks (50 g), at room temperature

1 teaspoon pure vanilla extract

¼ teaspoon pure almond extract

4 egg whites (100 g), at room temperature

Icing

8 tablespoons (112 g) unsalted butter, at room temperature

1½ cups (173 g) confectioners' sugar

¼ cup Butterscotch Sauce (see page 142), plus more as needed

---

yolks, and vanilla and almond extracts, whisking vigorously to combine well after each addition. In the bowl of a stand mixer fitted with the whisk attachment, or a large bowl with a hand mixer, whip the egg whites on medium-high speed until stiff (but not dry) peaks form. Add about half of the egg whites to the bowl of batter, and whisk to combine. Add the remaining egg whites, and carefully fold until no white streaks remain. Pour the batter into the prepared pan and spread it gently into an even layer.

Place the pan in the center of the preheated oven and bake, rotating the pan once, until the cake is nicely puffed and uniformly golden brown and has begun to pull away from the sides of the pan, about 30 minutes. Remove the pan from the oven and allow the cake to cool for 10 minutes in the pan before transferring to a wire rack set over a piece of parchment or waxed paper to cool completely.

While the cake cools, prepare the icing: In the clean bowl of a stand mixer fitted with the paddle attachment, or a large bowl with a hand mixer, place the butter and beat on high speed until light and fluffy. Add the confectioners' sugar, and mix on low speed until just combined. Drizzle in the ¼ cup of butterscotch sauce and continue to beat, adding more sauce by the tablespoon until the mixture is very light brown in color and smells and tastes of butterscotch. The icing should be thickly pourable.

With the cooled cake still on the rack, pour the icing in the center of the cake. With a small offset spatula, slowly and carefully spread the icing thickly over the top of the cake. Refrigerate until the icing has set and is nearly dry to the touch. With a very sharp knife, slice the cake into nine rectangular pieces. To achieve the traditional zigzag shape along the sides of the cakes, on each long side of the rectangles, gently use a small cookie cutter to cut two half-moons. Serve with extra butterscotch sauce for dipping.

These snack cakes are best enjoyed within 2 days of being iced, but they will keep for up to a month wrapped individually in freezer-safe wrap and frozen. Defrost at room temperature.

Tastykake Peanut Butter Kandy Kakes

MAKES 30 INDIVIDUAL CAKES

Kandy Kakes come in every sort of variety (mint! dark chocolate coconut!), but according to my bona fide Philadelphian husband, peanut butter Kandy Kakes are the standard. And about the name . . . Although even the Tastykake website makes a passing reference to their also being known as "Tandy Kakes," my husband thinks it's just a misnomer. Are those fightin' words? I hope not! These tender miniature sponge cakes with a layer of peanut butter crème, covered in chocolate, should bring us together, not drive us apart.

Prepare the cakes: Preheat your oven to 350°F. Grease the wells of a standard twelve-cup muffin tin and set the tin aside.

In a large bowl, place the flour blend, xanthan gum, cornstarch, baking powder, baking soda, salt, and granulated sugar, and whisk to combine well. Set the bowl of dry ingredients aside. In the bowl of a stand mixer fitted with the whisk attachment, or a large bowl with a hand mixer, place the two egg whites and beat on medium speed until stiff (but not dry) peaks form. Still using the whisk attachment, beat in the egg yolk and butter on medium speed. The mixture will be thick and the egg whites will deflate a bit, but the mixture will still be fluffy. Add the dry ingredients and the milk, alternating one and then the other, and beginning and ending with the dry ingredients. Mix until just combined. The batter will be pale yellow and light.

Fill the prepared muffin cups about one-quarter full, and place in the center of the preheated oven. Bake until the small cakes are pale golden and beginning to pull away from the sides of the pan, and a toothpick inserted into the center of a cake comes out clean, 10 to 12 minutes. Remove from the oven and allow to cool in the pan for at least 10 minutes before inverting the cakes onto a wire rack to cool completely. Position the wire rack over a piece of parchment or waxed paper.

Cakes

1¾ cups (245 g) basic gum-free gluten-free flour blend (see page 7)

¼ teaspoon xanthan gum

2 tablespoons (18 g) cornstarch

1 teaspoon baking powder

½ teaspoon baking soda

½ teaspoon kosher salt

1 cup (200 g) granulated sugar

2 egg whites (50 g, weighed out of shell) plus 1 egg yolk (25 g), at room temperature

8 tablespoons (112 g) unsalted butter, at room temperature

⅔ cup (5⅓ fluid ounces) milk

Filling

Peanut Butter Filling (page 110)

CONTINUED ON PAGE 146

CONTINUED FROM PAGE 145

Chocolate Glaze

16 ounces milk chocolate, chopped

4 tablespoons (56 g) virgin coconut oil

Prepare the Peanut Butter Filling. Once the cakes have cooled completely, spread about 1 tablespoon of the filling into an even layer on top of each cake, and allow to set at room temperature for about 10 minutes. The filling should harden a bit.

Prepare the glaze: In a small, heat-safe bowl, melt the chocolate and coconut oil according to the instructions on page 21. Allow the chocolate to sit at room temperature until it begins to thicken a bit. Place the cakes, one at a time, peanut butter side down, in the glaze. Press down on the cake with the tines of a fork, then flip it gently in the chocolate. Pull the cake out of the chocolate by slipping the fork under it and bobbing it on the surface of the chocolate a few times before pulling it along the edge of the bowl and carefully placing it on a clean sheet of waxed or parchment paper. Allow the chocolate glaze to set at room temperature.

These snack cakes are best enjoyed within 2 days of being glazed, but they will keep for up to a month wrapped individually in freezer-safe wrap and frozen. Defrost at room temperature. The chocolate coating may bloom a bit over time, but it won't affect the taste at all.

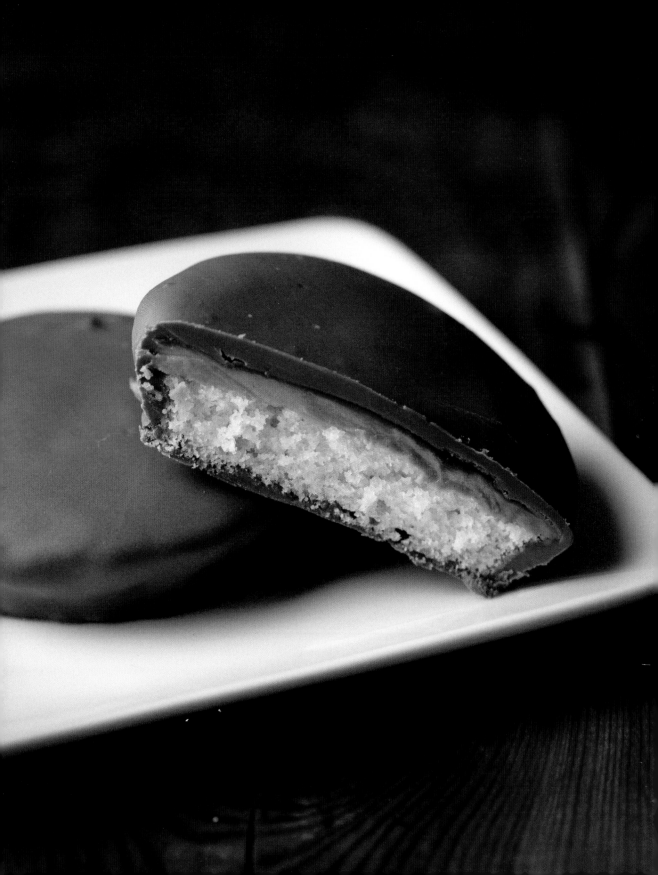

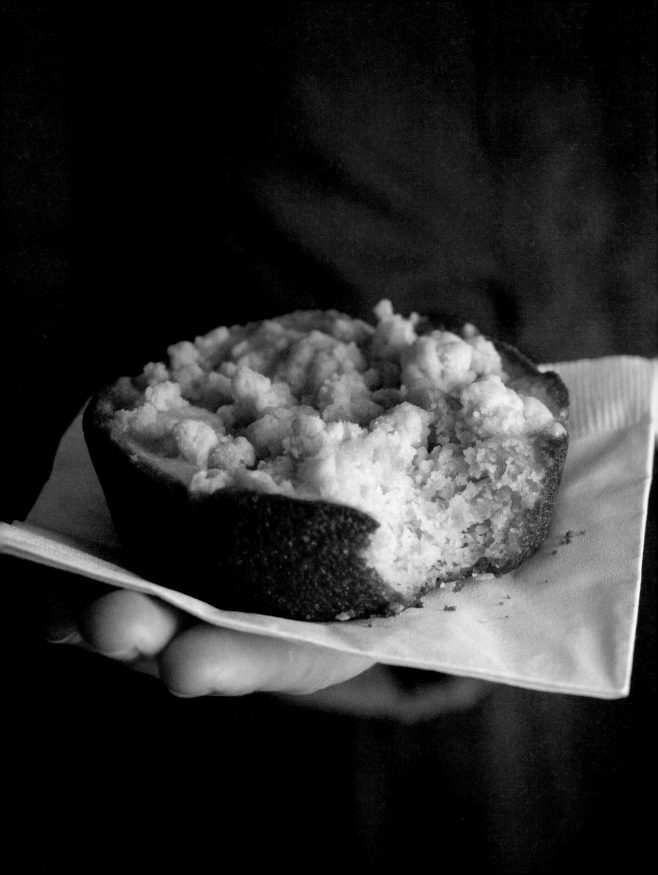

Drake's Coffee Cakes

MAKES 6 CAKES

*D*rake's Coffee Cakes are so tender and delicious that Jerry Seinfeld even attempts to use one as currency to buy off Newman in the third season of *Seinfeld* (until Elaine, who hasn't eaten in two days, steals and devours it). These moist and tender buttermilk cakes have at least as much sweet crumble topping as cake, so each bite has plenty of both. I bake them in a USA Pans Mini Round Cake Panel Pan, which has six wells, each 4 inches wide and about 1¼ inches deep. But if you don't have a specialty pan, these can easily be made as mini coffee cakes in a standard twelve-cup muffin tin. Just reduce the baking time as indicated in the recipe instructions.

Preheat your oven to 350°F. Grease the wells of a miniature cake panel pan (or a standard twelve-cup muffin tin) and set it aside.

First, prepare the crumble topping, as it has to be chilled until firm: In a medium-size bowl, place the flour, cornstarch, salt, and granulated sugar and whisk to combine well. Add the brown sugar and whisk again to combine, working out any lumps. Create a well in the center of the dry ingredients and add the butter and 2 tablespoons of the water. Mix until the topping holds together, add more water by the half-teaspoonful until it holds together. Cover the bowl with a piece of plastic wrap and place in the refrigerator to chill until firm, about 30 minutes.

While the topping is chilling, prepare the cakes: In a large bowl, place the flour, cornstarch, baking powder, baking soda, salt, and granulated sugar, and whisk to combine well. Add the brown sugar, and whisk again, working out any lumps. Create a well in the center of the dry ingredients and add the butter, shortening, eggs, egg white, buttermilk, and vanilla, mixing to combine after each addition. Fill each prepared well about halfway with cake batter. Remove the chilled topping from the refrigerator, and break it up into irregular pieces with the tines of a fork. Divide

Crumble Topping

1½ cups (210 g) all-purpose gluten-free flour (see page 2)

¼ cup (36 g) cornstarch

⅛ teaspoon kosher salt

⅓ cup (67 g) granulated sugar

⅓ cup (73 g) packed light brown sugar

8 tablespoons (112 g) unsalted butter, melted

2 to 3 tablespoons (1 to 1½ fluid ounces) lukewarm water

Cakes

1 cup (140 g) all-purpose gluten-free flour (see page 2)

¼ cup (36 g) cornstarch

¾ teaspoon baking powder

¼ teaspoon baking soda

¼ teaspoon kosher salt

CONTINUED ON PAGE 150

CONTINUED FROM PAGE 149

¾ cup (150 g) granulated sugar

3 tablespoons (40 g) packed light brown sugar

2 tablespoons (28 g) unsalted butter, at room temperature

4 tablespoons (48 g) nonhydrogenated vegetable shortening, melted and cooled

2 eggs (100 g, weighed out of shell) plus 1 egg white (25 g), at room temperature, beaten

½ cup (4 fluid ounces) buttermilk, at room temperature

1 teaspoon pure vanilla extract

———————

the pieces of the crumble topping among the wells half-filled with cake batter, and press gently to help the topping adhere to the cakes during baking.

Place the pan in the center of the preheated oven and bake until a toothpick inserted into the center of a cake comes out clean, about 20 minutes if using a panel pan (or 16 minutes for a muffin tin). Allow the cakes to cool for 10 minutes in the pan before transferring to a wire rack to cool completely.

These cakes will keep in a sealed plastic or glass container at room temperature for up to 3 days. For longer storage, seal them tightly in a freezer-safe wrap or bag, and freeze for up to 2 months. Defrost at room temperature.

Drake's Devil Dogs

MAKES 10 SNACK CAKES

I tried several variations on this recipe for Devil Dogs before I settled on the version you see before you. It was a sort of Goldilocks experience, if what Goldilocks was looking for was snack cakes with exactly the proper texture. This recipe is, hands down, the winner. The cakes are very chocolaty and the filling is rather stiff and not overly sweet, but more important, they stick to the roof of your mouth when you eat them. If you have no experience with this particular snack cake, that might sound like a bad thing. But if you are nostalgic for Devil Dogs, you're in for a rush. For the filling, I prefer the smoother texture of the 7-Minute Crème Filling for Snack Cakes, but the Stabilized Whipped Cream is also lovely.

Prepare the cakes: Preheat your oven to 350°F. Line rimmed baking sheets with unbleached parchment paper and set them aside.

In a medium-size bowl, place the flour, cornstarch, cocoa powder, baking soda, baking powder, and salt, and whisk to combine well. Set the bowl aside. In the bowl of a stand mixer fitted with the paddle attachment, or a large bowl with a hand mixer, beat the butter and shortening on medium-high speed until light and fluffy. Add the brown sugar, eggs, egg white, and vanilla, and beat on medium-high speed to combine after each addition. Add the dry ingredients and the milk alternately, beginning and ending with the dry ingredients, mixing on medium speed until well combined. The batter will be thick. Transfer it to a large pastry bag fitted with a ½-inch plain piping tip, and pipe 3½-inch-long cylinders 2 inches apart from one another on the prepared baking sheets. With wet fingers, press down firmly but carefully on each to flatten the tops and round the sides.

Place the baking sheets, one at a time, in the center of the preheated oven and bake for 10 minutes, or until the cakes spring back when

Cakes

1⅜ cup (193 g) all-purpose gluten-free flour (see page 2)

5½ tablespoons (50 g) cornstarch

⅔ cup (53 g) unsweetened cocoa powder

1 teaspoon baking soda

½ teaspoon baking powder

½ teaspoon kosher salt

4 tablespoons (56 g) unsalted butter, at room temperature

4 tablespoons (48 g) nonhydrogenated vegetable shortening

1 cup (218 g) packed light brown sugar

2 eggs (100 g, weighed out of shell) plus 1 egg white (25 g), at room temperature, beaten

CONTINUED ON PAGE 152

CONTINUED FROM PAGE 151

**1½ teaspoons pure
vanilla extract**

**1 cup (8 fluid ounces)
milk, at room temperature**

Filling

**7-Minute Crème Filling for
Snack Cakes (page 169)
or Stabilized Whipped
Cream for Snack Cakes
(page 170)**

———

pressed lightly in center. Remove from the oven and allow to cool for 10 minutes on the baking sheets before transferring to a wire rack to cool completely.

While the cakes are cooling, prepare the 7-Minute Crème Filling or Stabilized Whipped Cream. Invert half of the cooled cakes on a flat surface lined with parchment or waxed paper, then spread about ½ inch of filling on top, and cover each with another cake, right-side up. Press down gently to form a sandwich.

These snack cakes are best enjoyed the day they are made, but they will keep for up to a month wrapped individually in freezer-safe wrap and frozen. Defrost at room temperature.

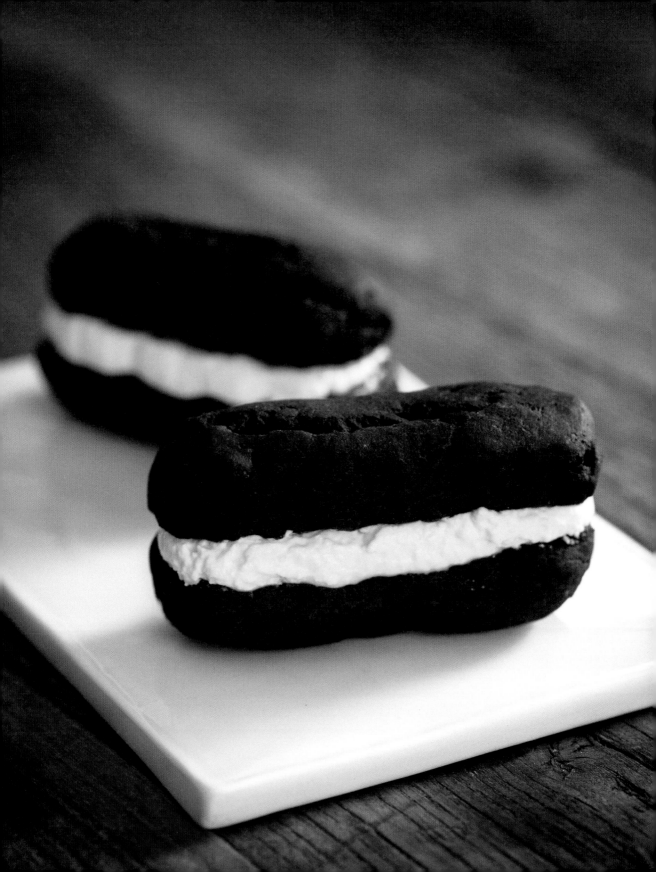

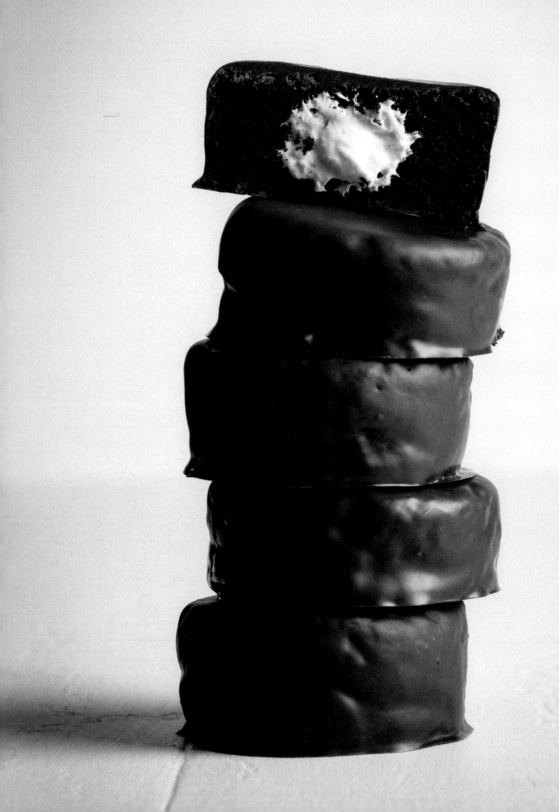

Drake's Ring Dings

MAKES 12 SNACK CAKES

rake's Ring Dings (or Hostess Ding Dongs) have a moist, dense devil's food–style cake with a smooth, creamy filling, all covered in a thick layer of rich chocolate glaze. While I was growing up, they were always my favorite chocolate snack cake. In these snack cakes, although you have a choice, I prefer the lighter texture of the Stabilized Whipped Cream for Snack Cakes. A couple of companies make the special pans for homemade snack cakes like Ring Dings, including Wilton (theirs is called a 12-Cavity Spool Cake Pan) and Fat Daddio (theirs is called a Choco Creme Snack Cake Pan or a Classic Chocolate-Covered Wheel Cupcake pan). But a standard twelve-cup muffin tin works perfectly well. In fact, Nordic Ware makes a standard twelve-cup aluminum muffin tin with wells that are relatively straight-sided. They'd make lovely home-made Ring Dings.

Prepare the cakes: Preheat your oven to 350°F. Grease twelve single-serving wells of an appropriate snack cake pan (or a standard twelve-cup muffin tin) and set it aside.

In the bowl of a stand mixer fitted with the paddle attachment, or a large bowl with a hand mixer, place the butter and beat on medium-high speed until light and fluffy. Add the sugar, eggs, sour cream, and vanilla, beating to combine after each addition. In a small bowl, place the flour, cocoa powder, baking soda, and salt, and whisk to combine well. Add the dry ingredients and water to the bowl of wet ingredients alternately, beginning and ending with the dry ingredients and mixing to combine well after each addition. Pour the batter into the prepared the pan, filling the wells two-thirds full.

Place the pan in the center of the preheated oven and bake until a toothpick inserted into the center of a cake comes out mostly clean,

Cakes

8 tablespoons (112 g) unsalted butter, at room temperature

1½ cups (327 g) packed light brown sugar

2 eggs (100 g, weighed out of shell), at room temperature

½ cup (120 g) sour cream, at room temperature

1 teaspoon pure vanilla extract

2 cups (280 g) all-purpose gluten-free flour (see page 2)

¾ cup (60 g) unsweetened cocoa powder

1¼ teaspoons baking soda

½ teaspoon kosher salt

1⅓ cups (10⅔ fluid ounces) warm water

CONTINUED ON PAGE 156

CONTINUED FROM PAGE 155

──────────

Filling

Stabilized Whipped Cream for Snack Cakes (page 170) or 7-Minute Crème Filling for Snack Cakes (page 169)

Chocolate Glaze

16 ounces semisweet chocolate, chopped

4 tablespoons (56 g) virgin coconut oil

──────────

13 to 15 minutes. Allow to cool in the pan for about 10 minutes before removing them. Slice off the rounded top of each cake to make a flat top and place on a wire rack, cut-side down, to cool completely.

While the cakes are cooling, prepare the Stabilized Whipped Cream or 7-Minute Crème Filling. Once the cakes have cooled, create a well in the center of the cut side of each cake with a ¾-inch round cookie cutter, cutting off the bottom with a knife (reserve the removed cake pieces). Transfer the filling to a pastry bag fitted with a ¼-inch plain piping tip and pipe about 1½ tablespoons of filling into the open well in each cake. Cover the filling in each cake with a previously removed cake piece. Invert the cakes and place them back on the wire rack, placed over a piece of parchment or waxed paper. Line a rimmed baking sheet with parchment or waxed paper and set it aside.

Prepare the glaze: In a small, heat-safe bowl, melt the chocolate and coconut oil for the glaze according to the instructions on page 21. Allow the chocolate to sit at room temperature until it begins to thicken a bit. Immerse the filled snack cakes, one at a time, in the glaze: Press down on the cake with the tines of a fork, then flip it gently in the chocolate. Pull the cake out of the chocolate by slipping the fork under it and bobbing it on the surface of the chocolate a few times before pulling it along the edge of the bowl and carefully placing it on the prepared baking sheet. Allow the chocolate glaze to set at room temperature.

These snack cakes are best enjoyed within 2 days of being glazed, but they will keep for up to a month wrapped individually in freezer-safe wrap and frozen. Defrost at room temperature. The chocolate coating may bloom a bit over time, but it won't affect the taste at all.

Drake's Sunny Doodles

MAKES 18 CUPCAKES

Hostess Chocolate Cupcakes (page 131), with their crème filling and distinctive frosting, are an icon. But what of the Sunny Doodle, an unfrosted (yet no less delicious) crème-filled cake? A very moist yellow cake, with delicious crème filling that pokes out the very top, this is your reprieve from the extra steps of some of the other snack cakes. Either of the recommended fillings will do, but I have a slight preference for the lighter Stabilized Whipped Cream for Snack Cakes here. Enjoy!

Prepare the cupcakes: Preheat your oven to 350°F. Line a standard twelve-cup muffin tin with cupcake liners or grease the wells and set the tin aside.

In a large bowl, place the flour, baking powder, baking soda, salt, and sugar, and whisk to combine well. Add the butter, eggs, vanilla, and milk, mixing to combine after each addition. The batter will be pourable.

Fill the prepared muffin cups about two-thirds full. Place the pan in the center of the preheated oven and bake until the cupcakes are lightly golden brown and a toothpick inserted into the center of a cupcake comes out with no more than a few moist crumbs attached, about 19 minutes. Allow the cupcakes to cool for at least 5 minutes in the tin before transferring to a wire rack to cool completely. Repeat with the remaining cupcake batter.

Meanwhile, prepare the Stabilized Whipped Cream or 7-Minute Crème Filling, and transfer it to a pastry bag fitted with a Bismarck tip.

Insert the pastry tip into the center of each cooled cupcake, wiggling it around a bit to create some space, then filling each with about 1½ tablespoons prepared filling. Be sure to fill enough that a bit of filling peeks out of the top of the cake.

These snack cakes are best enjoyed within 2 days of being filled, but they will keep for up to a month wrapped individually in freezer-safe wrap and frozen. Defrost at room temperature.

Cupcakes

1½ cups plus
2 tablespoons (228 g)
all-purpose gluten-free
flour (see page 2)

1 teaspoon baking powder

½ teaspoon baking soda

½ teaspoon kosher salt

1 cup (200 g) granulated
sugar

8 tablespoons (112 g)
unsalted butter, at room
temperature

2 eggs (100 g, weighed
out of shell), at room
temperature, beaten

2 teaspoons pure vanilla
extract

⅔ cup (5⅓ fluid
ounces) milk, at room
temperature

Filling

Stabilized Whipped
Cream for Snack Cakes
(page 170) or 7-Minute
Crème Filling for Snack
Cakes (page 169)

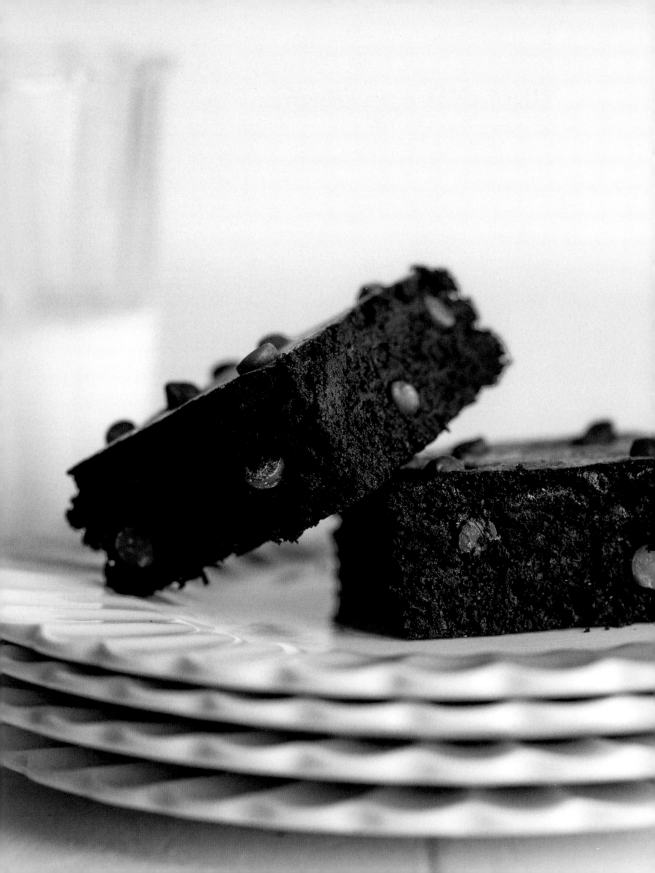

Weight Watchers Chocolate Brownies

MAKES 16 BROWNIES

These Weight Watchers brownies are, simply put, surprisingly good. The secret to their tender crumb might very well be that they're not fat free. There isn't a lot of fat in the recipe (less than 5 grams per brownie), but they have just enough of it to make them tender and delicious, without being overly sweet. Although both fat and sugar are tenderizers in baking, fat is more effective. That's why so many of the fat-free snack cakes from the 1990s were very, very sweet, but still a bit tough to chew. Weight Watchers has definitely changed with the times, and now we can finally keep pace! At only 3 PointsPlus points per brownie, there's no guilt.

Preheat your oven to 350°F. Grease and line a 9-inch square baking pan with two sheets of unbleached parchment paper, crisscrossed in the pan, with enough paper to overhang the edges, and set it aside.

In a large bowl, place the all-purpose flour, teff flour, cocoa powder, baking soda, salt, and sugar, and whisk to combine well. Create a well in the center of the dry ingredients and add the egg whites, corn syrup, and oil, mixing to combine after each addition. The batter will be thick. Add the cornstarch-dusted miniature chips, and mix until the chips are evenly distributed throughout the batter. Scrape the batter into the prepared pan and spread into an even layer.

Place the pan in the center of the preheated oven and bake until firm to the touch, about 15 minutes. Allow to cool for 10 minutes in the pan before lifting out of the pan by the parchment paper and transferring to a wire rack to cool completely. Once cool, slice into sixteen squares with a sharp knife.

The brownies can be stored in a sealed plastic or glass container at room temperature and should maintain their texture for at least 2 days. For longer storage, seal them tightly in a freezer-safe wrap or bag, and freeze for up to 2 months. Defrost at room temperature.

3 POINTSPLUS VALUE PER BROWNIE

⅓ cup (47 g) all-purpose gluten-free flour (see page 2)

¼ cup (30 g) teff flour

¾ cup (60 g) unsweetened cocoa powder

⅛ teaspoon baking soda

¼ teaspoon kosher salt

½ cup (100 g) granulated sugar

4 egg whites (100 g)

2 tablespoons (42 g) light corn syrup

¼ cup (56 g) canola oil

3 ounces miniature chocolate chips, tossed with ½ teaspoon cornstarch

Weight Watchers Lemon Crème Cakes

MAKES 8 CAKES

**3 POINTSPLUS
VALUE PER CAKE**

Cakes

**1¾ cups (245 g)
gluten-free cake flour
(see page 2)**

**3 tablespoons plus
1 teaspoon (20 g) nonfat
dry milk, ground into a
finer powder**

1 teaspoon baking powder

¼ teaspoon baking soda

¼ teaspoon kosher salt

**1 teaspoon finely grated
lemon zest**

**½ cup (100 g) granulated
sugar**

**4 tablespoons (56 g)
unsalted butter, at room
temperature**

**2 tablespoons (24 g)
nonhydrogenated
vegetable shortening,
melted and cooled**

CONTINUED ON PAGE 162

These zesty lemony little cakes are what would happen if Twinkies (page 129) slimmed down and brightened up with lemon zest and extract. They're not very large, but they aren't micro-minis, either. They're just the right size, in just the right, bright flavor. And just like their chocolate cousins (page 163), only 3 PointsPlus points.

Prepare the cakes: Preheat your oven to 350°F. Grease and line an 8-inch square pan with two sheets of unbleached parchment paper, crisscrossed in the pan, with enough paper to overhang the edges, and set it aside.

In a large bowl, place the cake flour, nonfat dry milk, baking powder, baking soda, salt, and lemon zest, and whisk to combine well, breaking up any clumps of lemon zest. Add the sugar, and whisk to combine. Create a well in the center of the dry ingredients, and add the butter, shortening, egg, egg whites, corn syrup, vanilla extract, lemon extract, and water, mixing to combine well after each addition. Scrape the batter into the prepared pan and smooth and shake into an even layer.

Place the pan in the center of the preheated oven and bake until the cake is very lightly golden brown and a toothpick inserted into the center comes out clean, about 22 minutes. Remove from the oven and allow to cool in the baking pan for 15 minutes before lifting out of the pan by the parchment paper and transferring to a wire rack to cool completely.

While the cake is cooling, prepare the filling: Place the cream cheese in the bowl of a stand mixer fitted with the paddle attachment, or a large bowl with a hand mixer, and beat on medium-high speed until light and fluffy. Add the confectioners' sugar, salt, lemon zest, and lemon extract, and mix on low speed until just combined. Raise the mixer speed to high, and beat until light and fluffy.

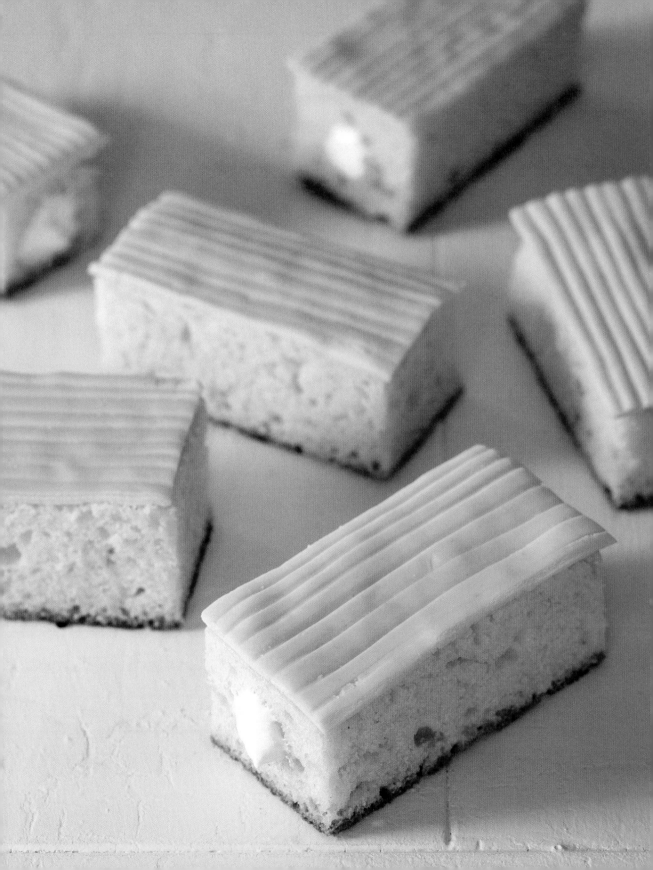

CONTINUED FROM PAGE 160

1 egg (50 g, weighed out of shell) plus 2 egg whites (50 g), at room temperature

2 tablespoons (42 g) light corn syrup

½ teaspoon pure vanilla extract

1 teaspoon pure lemon extract

½ cup (4 fluid ounces) lukewarm water

Crème Filling

6 ounces light (⅓ less fat) cream cheese, at room temperature

1¼ cups (144 g) confectioners' sugar

⅛ teaspoon kosher salt

½ teaspoon finely grated lemon zest

½ teaspoon pure lemon extract

Topping

Marshmallow Fondant (page 167)

Yellow food coloring (optional)

Once the cake is cool, slice with a sharp knife into 8 equal rectangles. Poke a wooden skewer or chopstick through each cake horizontally to create space for the filling. Transfer the filling to a pastry bag fitted with a Bismarck tip, and pipe filling into the cakes from both sides.

Prepare the topping: Prepare the Marshmallow Fondant. Knead the yellow food coloring, if using, into the fondant with your hands until you achieve a uniform color. Roll out the fondant to about ⅛ inch thick between two sheets of unbleached parchment paper and slice into rectangles about the size of each individual cake (about 2 x 4 inches). Using a wooden skewer, press lines into the top of each fondant rectangle to resemble its Weight Watchers prototype. Cover the top of each cake with a very thin layer of filling and top with a prepared piece of fondant. Press to adhere.

Once finished with fondant, these snack cakes are best enjoyed within 2 days. They will keep for up to a month wrapped individually in freezer-safe wrap and frozen, but the fondant may begin to dry out. Defrost at room temperature. Alternatively, freeze as filled without covering in fondant, and then top with fondant once defrosted.

Weight Watchers Chocolate Crème Cakes

MAKES 8 CAKES

Think of these Weight Watchers Chocolate Crème Cakes as the diet-friendly version of chocolate Twinkies. These rich chocolate cakes with the smooth chocolate crème filling, topped with chocolate fondant, don't sacrifice on flavor or texture even though they only have 3 Weight Watchers PointsPlus points each. They're just the little indulgence we need sometimes!

Prepare the cakes: Preheat your oven to 350°F. Grease and line an 8-inch square pan with two sheets of unbleached parchment paper, crisscrossed in the pan, with enough paper to overhang the edges, and set it aside.

In a medium-size, heat-safe bowl, place the butter and chocolate and melt as instructed on page 21. Add the sugar, corn syrup, and vanilla, mixing to combine well after each addition. Add the egg, egg whites, and water, mixing again to combine well. Set the bowl aside. In a separate large bowl, place the cake flour, cocoa powder, nonfat dry milk, baking powder, baking soda, and salt, and whisk to combine well. Create a well in the center of the dry ingredients, and add the wet ingredients, mixing to combine. Scrape the batter into the prepared pan and smooth and shake into an even layer.

Place in the center of the preheated oven and bake until a toothpick inserted into the center of the cake comes out clean, about 22 minutes. Remove from the oven and allow to cool in the baking pan for 15 minutes before lifting out of the pan by the parchment paper and transferring to a wire rack to cool completely.

While the cake is cooling, prepare the filling: Place the cream cheese in the bowl of a stand mixer fitted with the paddle attachment, or a large bowl with a hand mixer, and beat on medium-high speed until light and fluffy. Add the confectioners' sugar, cocoa powder, and salt, and mix on low speed until just combined. Raise the mixer speed to high, and beat until light and fluffy.

---

3 POINTSPLUS VALUE PER CAKE

Cakes

4 tablespoons (56 g) unsalted butter, chopped

2 ounces unsweetened chocolate, chopped

½ cup (100 g) granulated sugar

2 tablespoons (42 g) light corn syrup

2 teaspoons pure vanilla extract

1 egg (50 g, weighed out of shell) plus 2 egg whites (50 g), at room temperature

½ cup (4 fluid ounces) lukewarm water

1½ cups (210 g) gluten-free cake flour (see page 2)

½ cup (40 g) unsweetened cocoa powder

CONTINUED ON PAGE 165

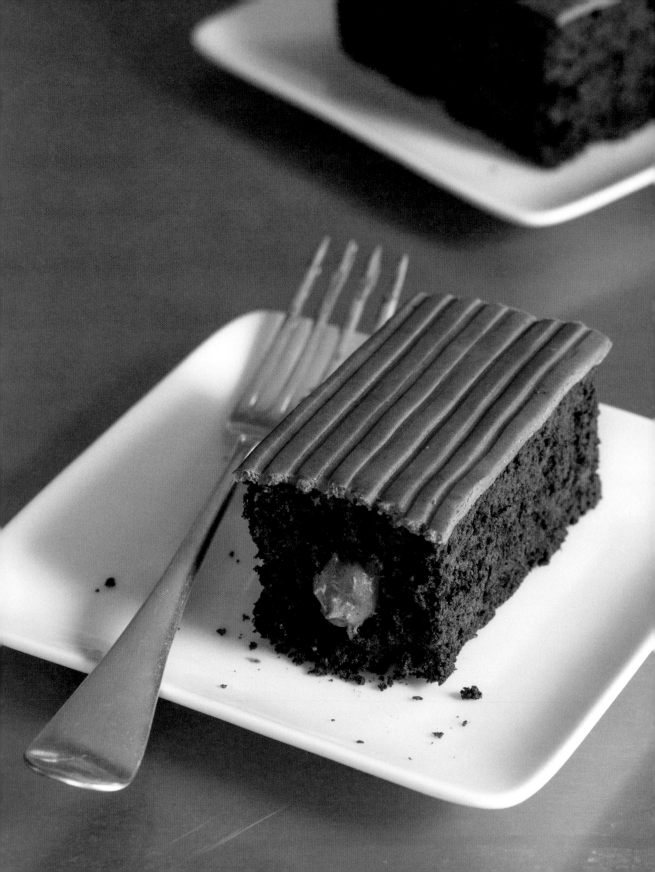

Once the cake is cool, slice with a sharp knife into eight equal rectangles. Poke a wooden skewer or chopstick through each cake horizontally to create space for the filling. Transfer the filling to a pastry bag fitted with a Bismarck tip, and pipe the filling into the cakes from both sides.

Prepare the topping: Prepare the Marshmallow Fondant. Knead the cocoa powder and food coloring, if using, into the fondant with your hands until you achieve a uniform color. Roll out the fondant to about 1/8 inch thick between two sheets of unbleached parchment paper and slice into rectangles about the size of each individual cake (about 2 x 4 inches). Using a wooden skewer, press lines into the top of each fondant rectangle to resemble its Weight Watchers prototype. Cover the top of each cake with a very thin layer of filling and top with a prepared piece of fondant. Press to adhere.

Once finished with fondant, these snack cakes are best enjoyed within 2 days. They will keep for up to a month wrapped individually in freezer-safe wrap and frozen, but the fondant may begin to dry out. Defrost at room temperature. Alternatively, freeze as filled without covering in fondant, and then top with fondant once defrosted.

CONTINUED FROM PAGE 163

3 tablespoons plus
1 teaspoon (20 g) nonfat
dry milk, ground into a
finer powder

1 teaspoon baking powder

1/4 teaspoon baking soda

1/4 teaspoon kosher salt

Crème Filling

6 ounces light (1/3 less
fat) cream cheese, at
room temperature

1 cup (115 g)
confectioners' sugar

1/4 cup (20 g)
unsweetened cocoa
powder

1/8 teaspoon kosher salt

Topping

Marshmallow Fondant
(page 167)

2 teaspoons (10 g)
unsweetened cocoa
powder

Brown food coloring
(optional)

Marshmallow Fluff

MAKES ABOUT 3 CUPS FLUFF

1¼ cups (250 g) granulated sugar

½ cup (4 fluid ounces) water

⅛ teaspoon kosher salt

2 egg whites (50 g), at room temperature

⅛ teaspoon cream of tartar

1 teaspoon pure vanilla extract

*H*ere's a little secret: You could actually use Marshmallow Fluff as the filling in all the snack cakes in Chapter 3. Make up a big batch, and you can store it in the refrigerator for at least two days and it will stay fresh. Fluff is sort of like marshmallows, but the stabilizer is egg whites instead of gelatin. It has a nice, light texture and flavor and is delicious served on top of cake or ice cream. Homemade fluff keeps rather well in the refrigerator for at least two days, but the sugars begin to crystallize by the third day. It does not freeze well on its own, but it freezes fine when used as a filling in snack cakes.

In a medium-size, heavy-bottomed saucepan, place the sugar, water, and salt, and whisk to combine. Clip a candy thermometer to the side of the saucepan and cook the sugar mixture over medium-high heat, without stirring it, until it reaches 240°F. Remove from the heat and set it aside to cool briefly.

Place the egg whites in the bowl of a stand mixer fitted with the whisk attachment, or a large bowl with a hand mixer. Whip the egg whites on medium-high speed until beginning to thicken. Add the cream of tartar and vanilla, and continue to whip until stiff (but not dry) peaks form. With the mixer speed on low, pour the warm sugar mixture down the side of the mixer (making sure the sugar doesn't hit the whisk). Once all the sugar mixture has been added, raise the mixer speed to high and beat until the mixture is thick, glossy, and at least doubled in size, and holds a stiff peak, about 5 minutes.

Marshmallow Fondant

MAKES ABOUT 1 POUND FONDANT

*F*ondant is the reason some cakes look impossibly smooth and finished. It's the peel-off sort of icing that can be made any color of the rainbow with enough gel food coloring, and it can transform a cake into a spaceship or a wrapped present and everything in between. Marshmallow fondant is the easiest sort of fondant to make at home, and it's also delicious to eat, unlike store-bought fondant. To make authentic-looking Weight Watchers Crème Cakes (pages 160–163), you'll need to make fondant. If you have never worked with fondant before, you might be intimidated by the thought. Well, you'll be amazed by how easy fondant is to make and to work with. It can also be made days and days ahead of time, wrapped tightly in plastic wrap and stored at room temperature. I have made it up to seven days before using it and never had a problem.

7 ounces store-bought gluten-free marshmallows (Kraft and Campfire brands are gluten-free in the United States as of the printing of this book)

1 tablespoon (½ fluid ounce) lukewarm water

1 teaspoon freshly squeezed lemon juice

1 teaspoon (7 g) light corn syrup

¼ teaspoon kosher salt

3 to 4 cups (345 to 460 g) confectioners' sugar

Spray a medium-size, microwave-safe bowl with cooking oil spray and place the marshmallows and water in the bowl. Microwave at 70% power for 30 seconds at a time, stirring between intervals, until the marshmallows are melted enough to have a soupy consistency. Remove from the microwave and add the lemon juice, corn syrup, and salt, and mix to combine well. Set the bowl aside.

Spray the bowl and dough hook attachment of a stand mixer with cooking oil spray, or prepare a large bowl with a hand mixer fitted with the dough hook attachments. Place 3 cups of the confectioners' sugar in the bowl. Create a well in the center of the confectioners' sugar and pour in the marshmallow mixture. Knead the mixture on low speed until the wet ingredients have been incorporated into the sugar, about 2 minutes. The mixture will begin to stick to the bowl. Touch the fondant. It should have the consistency of modeling clay (pliable and not overly stiff but readily holds its shape when molded). Add more confectioners' sugar as necessary to achieve the desired consistency. Knead the fondant with greased hands until it is smooth. If you do not have any sort of mixer with dough hooks, you can make the fondant with well-oiled hands from start to finish, but it will be much harder and much messier!

Turn out the fondant onto a large piece of plastic wrap and wrap very tightly. Place in a resealable plastic bag, press out all the air and seal tightly. Allow the fondant to rest covered like that at room temperature for at least a few hours before working with it. Store the fondant as is until you are ready to use it, at which point you can knead in any flavors or food colorings as directed in an individual recipe.

This fondant can be made up to a week ahead of time with good results.

7-Minute Crème Filling for Snack Cakes

MAKES ABOUT 3 CUPS FROSTING

This frosting is so-named because, after bringing the mixture to 160°F over indirect heat, it takes seven minutes to beat with a whisk into a light and fluffy frosting. It's the simplest frosting, is stable at room temperature, and is quite similar to Marshmallow Fluff (page 166), differing mostly in method and proportion of ingredients. Used as a snack cake filling, it is a bit more dense than the Stabilized Whipped Cream for Snack Cakes (page 170), but they are very similar. It will keep reasonably well in a sealed container in the refrigerator for two days, after which it may begin to separate.

Place all the ingredients in the bowl of a stand mixer, or a large heat-safe bowl to use with a hand mixer, and whisk together to combine well. Place the bowl over a simmering pot of water, making sure the water doesn't touch the mixing bowl, and cook until the mixture reaches 160°F on an instant-read thermometer, about 4 minutes. Remove from the heat and beat with the whisk attachment (or a hand mixer) on medium-high speed until light and fluffy, about 7 minutes.

1½ cups (300 g) granulated sugar

½ teaspoon cream of tartar

¼ cup (2 fluid ounces) lukewarm water

3 egg whites (75 g), at room temperature

Stabilized Whipped Cream for Snack Cakes

MAKES ABOUT 4 CUPS WHIPPED CREAM

1 tablespoon (7 g) unflavored powdered gelatin

¼ cup (2 fluid ounces) water

2 cups (16 fluid ounces) heavy whipping cream, chilled

2 tablespoons (14 g) confectioners' sugar

There are two secrets to making perfect homemade whipped cream: temperature and speed. The heavy whipping cream must be well chilled, and even the bowl you are whipping the cream in should be chilled, for best results. The speed of the stand mixer or hand mixer used to whip the cream should be medium (I turn my stand mixer to 4 and my 5-speed hand mixer to 3), which will create a more stable whipped cream. But the only way to create a whipped cream that is truly going to be stable enough to use as filling for snack cakes, and that will stay stable at room temperature, is to add some gelatin. Incorporating standard, heat-soluble powdered gelatin into fresh whipped cream can be a bit tricky, as the gelatin must be bloomed in water and then heated to melt. Simply allow the bloomed, melted gelatin to cool until it is no longer hot to the touch. It should incorporate into the whipped cream fully. However, if you are looking for the easiest way out, use cold-water-soluble powdered gelatin. Simply mix it into the water, as directed below, but do not heat it. It will dissolve completely in the water. Then, continue with the instructions as written. (See page 10 for more about gelatin.) This whipped cream can be made ahead of time and stored in the refrigerator for two to three days, at which point it may begin to separate a bit. It does not freeze well on its own, but it freezes fine when used as a filling in snack cakes.

If using heat-soluble powdered gelatin, bloom it by placing it and the water in a small, heat-safe bowl, and stirring it gently to combine. Allow the mixture to sit at room temperature until the gelatin swells. Place the gelatin mixture in the microwave and melt at 60% power for 20 seconds until melted. Set the gelatin aside to cool briefly. For cold-water soluble gelatin, simply place the same amount of gelatin and the water together in a small bowl, and stir gently to combine.

In the bowl of a stand mixer fitted with the whisk attachment, or a large bowl with a hand mixer, place the chilled cream and whisk on medium speed until soft peaks form. Add the confectioners' sugar, and beat until stiff, glossy peaks form. Add the cooled gelatin, and beat until thickened, about 3 minutes.

Royal Icing

2¼ teaspoons meringue powder

1 cups (115 g) confectioners' sugar, plus more if necessary

1 tablespoon (½ fluid ounce) lukewarm water, plus more if necessary

*W*e both know that you really, really would like to be able to pipe the *perfect* swirl on top of your Hostess Chocolate Cupcakes (page 131). You can use some extra snack cake filling and pipe it through a small pastry tip. But if you want the perfect, clean lines, royal icing it is. When adding water here, go slowly. As with all types of glaze, it is much easier to thin than to thicken. For royal icing, meringue powder is essential and has no substitute. The icing can be stored in an airtight container at room temperature for at least a week. Before using it, place back in your mixing bowl and beat, adding water by the drop as necessary to achieve the proper consistency.

In a the bowl of a stand mixer fitted with the paddle attachment, or a large bowl with a hand mixer, place all the ingredients and mix on low speed until the sugar is absorbed. Raise the mixer speed to medium, and beat until the beater leaves a visible trail in the icing, about 10 minutes. To thicken, beat at higher speed and for more time, and/or add more confectioners' sugar. To thin, add more water by the quarter-teaspoonful and beat to combine.

Royal icing will thicken as it stands, and it is best made right before you work with it. If it has thickened upon standing, add water by the quarter-teaspoonful and beat it on medium-high speed to reestablish the proper consistency.

CHAPTER 4

Crackers & Other Savory, Crunchy Snacks

Crispy, Crunchy, and Sometimes Buttery

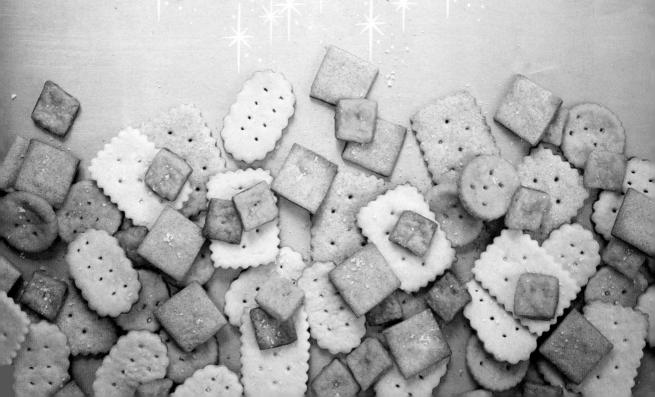

Keebler Town House Crackers, Original

MAKES ABOUT 50 CRACKERS

1¾ cups plus
2 tablespoons (263 g)
all-purpose gluten-free
flour (see page 2)

6 tablespoons (54 g)
cornstarch

7 tablespoons (42 g)
nonfat dry milk, ground
into a finer powder

½ teaspoon kosher salt,
plus more for sprinkling

½ teaspoon baking soda

¼ teaspoon baking
powder

2 tablespoons (25 g)
granulated sugar

10 tablespoons (140 g)
unsalted butter, at room
temperature

1 egg yolk (25 g), at room
temperature

6 to 8 tablespoons (3 to
4 fluid ounces) milk, at
room temperature

*L*argely the same as Original Keebler Club Crackers (page 176), these Town House crackers are cut thicker (and in a different shape—dramatic, I know). As sticklers will know, Town House Crackers do taste different: They are a bit saltier and slightly less sweet than their Club cousins.

Preheat your oven to 350°F. Line rimmed baking sheets with unbleached parchment paper and set them aside.

In a large bowl, place the flour, cornstarch, nonfat dry milk, the ¼ teaspoon of kosher salt, and the baking soda, baking powder, and sugar, and whisk to combine well. Create a well in the center of the dry ingredients and add the butter, egg yolk, and 3 fluid ounces of the milk, mixing to combine after each addition. Add more milk by the half-teaspoonful as necessary to hold the dough together.

Turn out the dough onto a lightly floured surface and roll out into an even layer about ¼ inch thick. The dough should roll out easily and will become smoother as you roll it out. Cut into 2½-inch-long scalloped rectangles and pierce randomly on top with a toothpick or wooden skewer. Place about 1 inch apart on the prepared baking sheets. Gather and reroll the scraps to cut out more crackers until you've used up the dough. Brush the tops of the raw crackers lightly with water, and sprinkle evenly with kosher salt.

Place the baking sheets, one at a time, in the center of the preheated oven and bake for 12 minutes, or until the crackers are very light golden brown all over. Allow to cool for 10 minutes on the baking sheets before transferring to a wire rack to cool completely.

The crackers can be stored in a sealed glass container at room temperature and should maintain their texture for at least 5 days. For longer storage, seal them tightly in a freezer-safe wrap or bag, and freeze for up to 2 months. Defrost at room temperature.

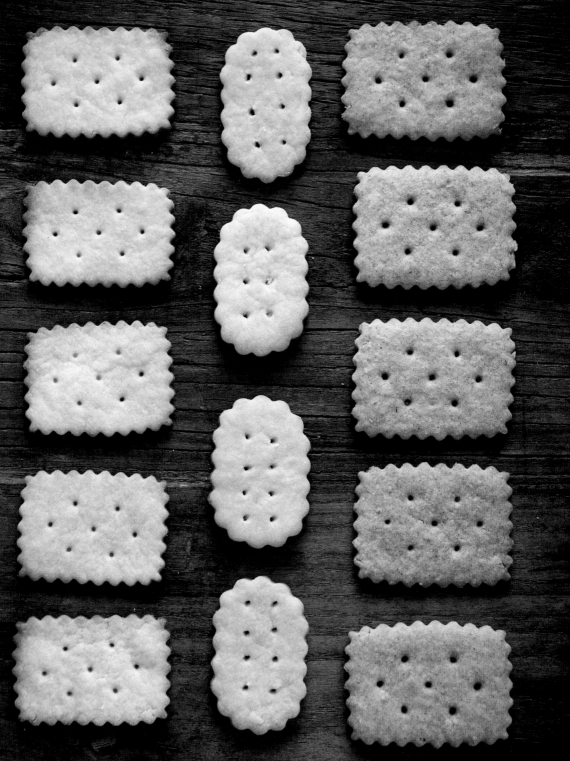

FROM LEFT TO RIGHT: Keebler Club Crackers, Original, page 176; Keebler Town House Crackers, Original, page 174; and Keebler Club Crackers, Multi-Grain, page 177

Keebler Club Crackers, Original

MAKES ABOUT 60 CRACKERS

1¾ cups plus
2 tablespoons (263 g)
all-purpose gluten-free
flour (see page 2), plus
more for sprinkling

6 tablespoons (54 g)
cornstarch

7 tablespoons (42 g)
nonfat dry milk, ground
into a finer powder

¼ teaspoon kosher salt,
plus more for sprinkling

½ teaspoon baking soda

¼ teaspoon baking
powder

3 tablespoons (38 g)
granulated sugar

10 tablespoons (140 g)
unsalted butter, at room
temperature

1 egg yolk (25 g), at room
temperature

6 to 8 tablespoons (3 to
4 fluid ounces) milk, at
room temperature

*I*n case you don't remember, Club Crackers are thin, crispy, and buttery, and they melt in your mouth. The sweetness is very subtle, as it should be. If you're too heavy-handed with the sugar, you'll find out (as I did along the way in developing this recipe) that they go from lovely to significantly less so.

Preheat your oven to 350°F. Line rimmed baking sheets with unbleached parchment paper and set them aside.

In a large bowl, place the flour, cornstarch, nonfat dry milk, the ¼ teaspoon of kosher salt, and the baking soda, baking powder, and sugar, and whisk to combine well. Create a well in the center of the dry ingredients and add the butter, egg yolk, and 3 fluid ounces of the milk, mixing to combine after each addition. Add more milk by the half-teaspoonful as necessary for the dough to hold together.

Turn out the dough onto a lightly floured surface and roll out into an even layer about ⅛ inch thick sprinkling lightly with flour as necessary. The dough should roll out easily and will become smoother as you roll it. Cut into 2¼-inch-long rectangles and pierce randomly on top with a toothpick or wooden skewer. Place about 1 inch apart on the prepared baking sheets. Gather and reroll the scraps to cut out more crackers until you've used up the dough. Brush the tops of the raw crackers lightly with water, and sprinkle evenly with kosher salt.

Place the baking sheets, one at a time, in the center of the preheated oven and bake for 10 minutes, or until the crackers are very light golden brown all over. Allow to cool for 10 minutes on the baking sheets before transferring to a wire rack to cool completely.

The crackers can be stored in a sealed glass container at room temperature and should maintain their texture for at least 5 days. For longer storage, seal them tightly in a freezer-safe wrap or bag, and freeze for up to 2 months. Defrost at room temperature.

Keebler Club Crackers, Multi-Grain

MAKES ABOUT 50 CRACKERS

The original Multi-Grain Club Crackers are, of course, made with wheat flour. To mimic the taste of whole wheat, I rely upon my tried-and-true blend of 75 percent sweet white sorghum flour and 25 percent teff flour. Combined with oat flour and all-purpose gluten-free flour, these key ingredients make for slightly nutty crackers that are a real treat.

Preheat your oven to 350°F. Line rimmed baking sheets with unbleached parchment paper and set them aside.

In a large bowl, place the flour, cornstarch, whole-grain flour blend, oat flour, nonfat dry milk, ¼ teaspoon of the kosher salt, and the baking soda, baking powder, and sugar, and whisk to combine well. Create a well in the center of the dry ingredients and add the butter, egg, and 1 fluid ounce of the water, mixing to combine after each addition. Add more water by the half-teaspoonful as necessary for the dough to hold together.

Turn out the dough onto a lightly floured surface and roll out into an even layer about ⅛ inch thick. The dough should roll out easily and will become smoother as you roll it. Cut into 2¼-inch-long rectangles and pierce randomly on top with a toothpick or wooden skewer. Place about 1 inch apart on the prepared baking sheets. Gather and reroll the scraps to cut out more crackers until you've used up the dough. Brush the tops of the raw crackers lightly with water, and sprinkle evenly with kosher salt.

Place the baking sheets, one at a time, in the center of the preheated oven and bake for 9 to 10 minutes, or until the crackers are very light golden brown all over. Allow to cool for 10 minutes on the baking sheets before transferring to a wire rack to cool completely.

The crackers can be stored in a sealed glass container at room temperature and should maintain their texture for at least 5 days. For longer storage, seal them tightly in a freezer-safe wrap or bag, and freeze for up to 2 months. Defrost at room temperature.

----

1 cup (140 g) all-purpose gluten-free flour (see page 2)

¼ cup (36 g) cornstarch

½ cup (70 g) whole-grain gluten-free flour blend (see page 8)

¼ cup (30 g) certified gluten-free oat flour

7 tablespoons (42 g) nonfat dry milk, ground into a finer powder

¼ teaspoon kosher salt, plus more for sprinkling

½ teaspoon baking soda

¼ teaspoon baking powder

¼ cup (50 g) granulated sugar

10 tablespoons (140 g) unsalted butter, at room temperature

1 egg (50 g, weighed out of shell), at room temperature

2 to 4 tablespoons (1 to 2 fluid ounces) water, at room temperature

----

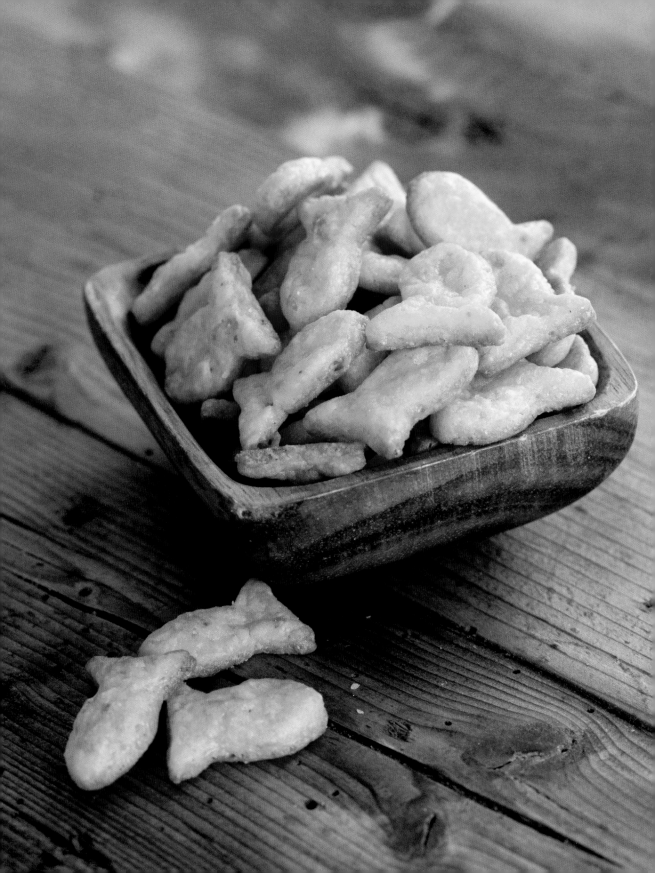

Pepperidge Farm Goldfish Baked Snack Crackers, Cheddar

MAKES ABOUT 70 CRACKERS

Pepperidge Farm now makes a gluten-free product called "Goldfish Puffs" that are something *like* the Goldfish we all know and love. But the delightfully crispy, crunchy, and cheesy crackers made with this recipe are much closer to the original Goldfish than the puffs. I sprung for the specialized miniature fish cookie cutter from CopperGifts.com (see Resources, page 295), but you could take any small aluminum cookie cutter and bend it into a simple fish shape, or just cut out 1½ x ¾-inch rectangles.

Preheat your oven to 350°F. Line rimmed baking sheets with unbleached parchment paper and set them aside.

Place all the ingredients, except the water, in the order listed, in the bowl of your food processor fitted with the steel blade. Add 2 tablespoons of the water and pulse, adding more water by the half-teaspoonful with the processor running, just until the dough comes together.

Turn out the dough onto a lightly floured surface and roll out into an even layer about ¼ inch thick sprinkling lightly with flour as necessary. The dough should roll out easily and will become smoother as you roll it. Cut out small goldfish shapes about 1½ inches in length and place about 1 inch apart from one another on the prepared baking sheets. Gather and reroll the scraps to cut out more crackers until you've used up the dough.

Place the baking sheets, one at a time, in the center of the preheated oven and bake for 10 to 12 minutes, or until the crackers are very light golden brown all over. They will crisp as they cool.

The crackers can be stored in a sealed glass container at room temperature and should maintain their texture for at least 5 days. For longer storage, seal them tightly in a freezer-safe wrap or bag, and freeze for up to 2 months. Defrost at room temperature.

---

1 cup (140 g) all-purpose gluten-free flour (see page 2), plus more for sprinkling

½ teaspoon kosher salt

⅛ teaspoon baking soda

⅛ teaspoon baking powder

½ teaspoon smoked Spanish paprika

4 tablespoons (56 g) cold unsalted butter, chopped

8 ounces shredded sharp yellow Cheddar cheese

2 to 4 tablespoons (1 to 2 fluid ounces) cold water

Wasabi Peas

MAKES ABOUT 4 CUPS WASABI PEAS

2 tablespoons (12 g) gluten-free wasabi powder (I used Eden brand)

¼ cup (36 g) basic gum-free gluten-free flour blend (see page 7)

2 tablespoons (18 g) cornstarch

2 teaspoons (8 g) granulated sugar

3 tablespoons (42 g) canola oil

1 teaspoon Dijon mustard

1 teaspoon white wine vinegar

½ cup (4 fluid ounces) lukewarm water, plus more by the teaspoonful

8 ounces freeze-dried peas

*T*he secret to making crunchy, savory, and spicy wasabi peas is to use freeze-dried peas. Luckily, freeze-dried fruits and vegetables are relatively easy to find in larger grocery stores (Just Tomatoes, Etc.! brand makes all manner of freeze-dried fruits and vegetables) and online at Nuts.com. Plus, it's much cheaper than buying a dehydrator. The peas will actually become a bit soggy when you first coat them in the wasabi paste, but they will crisp back up as they bake and cool again. They'll even stay crisp for a couple weeks in a sealed glass jar at room temperature.

Preheat your oven to 250°F. Line a half sheet (18 x 13 x 1-inch) pan with unbleached parchment paper and set it aside.

In a medium-size bowl, mix the wasabi powder, gum-free flour blend, cornstarch, and sugar in a small bowl, and whisk to combine well. Create a well in the center of the dry ingredients, and add the oil, mustard, and vinegar, mixing to combine after each addition. Add enough water to form a thick, soft paste. Add the freeze-dried peas to the bowl, and toss to coat.

Transfer to the prepared baking sheet, and, with wet hands, spread into an even layer. Place in the center of the preheated oven and bake for 15 minutes. Remove from the oven and stir to redistribute the peas. Return to the oven and continue to bake until crisp, another 10 to 15 minutes. Remove from the oven and allow to cool completely on the baking sheet. The peas will crisp as they cool.

The peas can be stored in a sealed glass container at room temperature and should maintain their texture for at least 7 days, perhaps even longer. Every once in a while when you pass by the container, give it a shake to ensure that the peas don't begin to stick to one another.

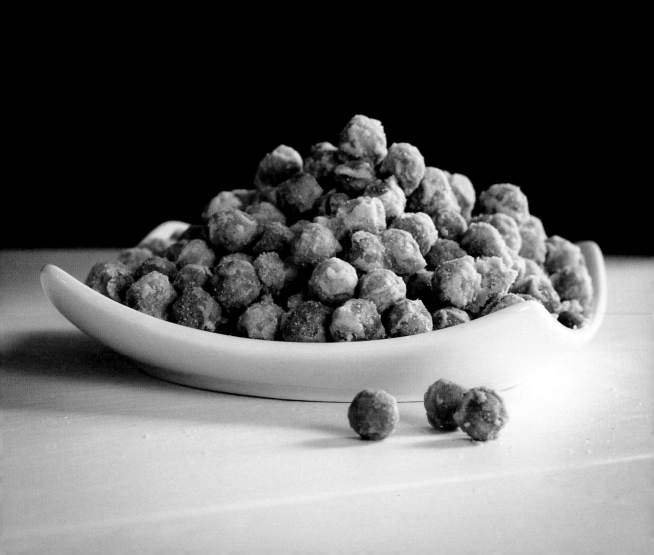

Nabisco Cheese Nips

1 cup plus 2 tablespoons (158 g) all-purpose gluten-free flour (see page 2), plus more for sprinkling

½ teaspoon kosher salt, plus more for sprinkling

⅛ teaspoon baking soda

½ teaspoon smoked Spanish paprika

4 tablespoons (56 g) cold unsalted butter, chopped

8 ounces shredded sharp yellow Cheddar cheese

2 to 4 tablespoons (1 to 2 fluid ounces) cold water

*I*f there is any real difference between Nabisco Cheese Nips and Sunshine Cheez-Its, I can't figure out what it is. Whichever brand name you prefer, these crispy, intensely cheesy little snacks are as addictive as you remember. The secret ingredient here? Paprika. And not just any old paprika, smoked Spanish paprika, for just a hint of that smoky flavor.

Preheat your oven to 350°F. Line rimmed baking sheets with unbleached parchment paper and set them aside.

Place all the ingredients, except the water, in the order listed, in the bowl of your food processor fitted with the steel blade. Add 2 tablespoons of the water and pulse, adding more water by the half-teaspoonful as necessary with the processor running, just until the dough comes together.

Turn out the dough onto a lightly floured surface and roll out into an even layer about ¼ inch thick sprinkling lightly with flour as necessary. The dough should roll out easily and will become smoother as you roll it. Cut into 1¼-inch squares with a square cookie cutter or a sharp knife, pizza wheel, or pastry wheel. Place the squares about 1 inch apart on the prepared baking sheets, and pierce one hole in the center of each with a toothpick or wooden skewer. Gather and reroll the scraps to cut out more crackers until you've used up the dough. Brush the tops of the raw crackers lightly with water, and sprinkle evenly with kosher salt.

Place the baking sheets, one at a time, in the center of the preheated oven and bake for 10 to 12 minutes, or until the crackers are very light golden brown all over. They will crisp as they cool.

The crackers can be stored in a sealed glass container at room temperature and should maintain their texture for at least 5 days. For longer storage, seal them tightly in a freezer-safe wrap or bag, and freeze for up to 2 months. Defrost at room temperature.

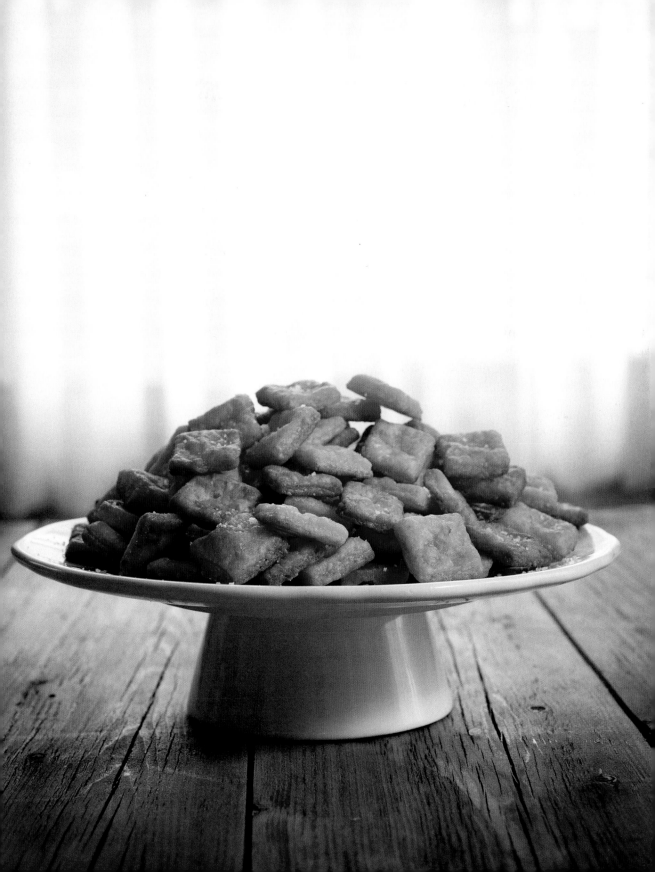

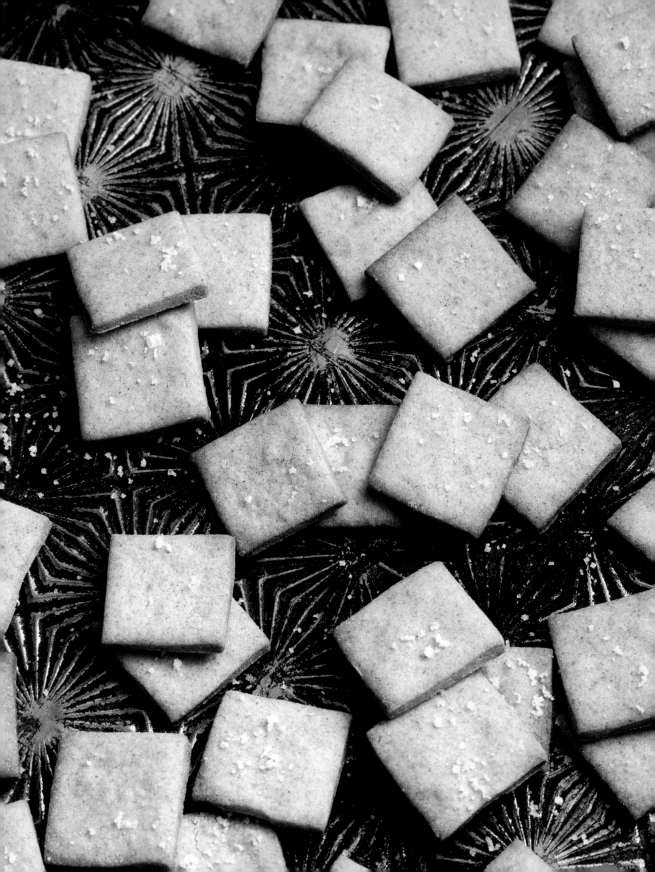

Nabisco Wheat Thins, Original

MAKES ABOUT 100 CRACKERS

W heat Thins are a sturdier cracker than the others in this chapter. I usually put quotation marks around the word *wheat*, as that term alone can strike fear in the heart of a trusting gluten-free person, who came here for delicious gluten-free recipes for their favorite cookies, crackers, and snack cakes. But I think by now, at this point in our relationship, you trust me not to include any actual wheat in the recipe, even without the quotes. My whole-grain flour blend, used to mimic the taste of whole wheat, is 75 percent sweet white sorghum flour, 25 percent teff flour, and 100 percent delicious. The sorghum flour adds protein and a touch of sweetness and chew, and the teff flour brings more protein, fiber, and a wheat-like color, too.

Preheat your oven to 350°F. Line rimmed baking sheets with unbleached parchment paper and set them aside.

In a large bowl, place the all-purpose flour, whole-grain flour blend, sugar, baking powder, baking soda, and 1 teaspoon of the kosher salt, and whisk to combine well. Create a well in the center of the dry ingredients, add the butter and milk, and mix to combine until the dough comes together. Knead until smooth. Divide the dough into two parts and press each into a small ball.

Place the first ball of dough between two sheets of unbleached parchment paper and roll with a rolling pin into a rectangle about ⅛ inch thick. The dough should roll out quickly and easily. With a sharp knife, pastry or pizza wheel, or a square cookie cutter, slice the dough into 1¼-inch squares. Place the squares 1 inch apart from one another on the prepared baking sheets. Gather and reroll the scraps to cut out more crackers until you've used up the dough. Repeat with the

---

1¼ cups (175 g)
all-purpose gluten-free
flour (see page 2)

¾ cup (105 g)
whole-grain gluten-free
flour blend (see page 8)

6 tablespoons (75 g)
granulated sugar

1½ teaspoons baking
powder

¼ teaspoon baking soda

1 teaspoon kosher salt,
plus more for sprinkling

6 tablespoons (84 g)
unsalted butter, melted
and cooled

½ cup (4 fluid
ounces) milk, at room
temperature

---

other half of dough. Sprinkle the tops of the squares generously with kosher salt.

Place the baking sheets, one at a time, in the center of the preheated oven and bake, rotating once halfway through baking, for about 9 minutes, or until the crackers are golden brown around the edges. Allow to cool completely on the baking sheets.

The crackers can be stored in a sealed glass container at room temperature and should maintain their texture for at least 5 days. For longer storage, seal them tightly in a freezer-safe wrap or bag, and freeze for up to 2 months. Defrost at room temperature.

Nabisco Premium Soup & Oyster Crackers

MAKES ABOUT 120 CRACKERS

*T*hinking about skipping the yeast in these oyster crackers? Be prepared for a heavier, denser cracker that just misses the mark. It's the combination of baking soda, baking powder, seltzer, *and* yeast that elevates these puffy little crackers to the status of soup and oyster crackers. If you don't have the tiny eight-sided cookie cutter to make the most authentic shape, ½-inch squares are fine.

Preheat your oven to 300°F. Line rimmed baking sheets with unbleached parchment paper and set them aside.

In a large bowl, place the flour, baking soda, baking powder, yeast, and sugar, and whisk to combine well. Add the ½ teaspoon of kosher salt and the cream of tartar, and whisk again to combine. Create a well in the center of the dry ingredients and add the shortening, butter, and 2 tablespoons seltzer, mixing to combine after each addition. Add more seltzer by the teaspoon as necessary to bring the dough together.

Transfer to a lightly floured surface and roll out to about ¼ inch thick. Cut out shapes with an eight-sided cutter that is about ¾ inch across, and place on the prepared baking sheets about 1½ inches apart. Gather and reroll the scraps to cut out more crackers until you've used up the dough. Cover with oiled plastic wrap and allow to sit for 40 minutes, or until beginning to swell. Brush the tops of the raw crackers lightly with water, and sprinkle evenly with kosher salt.

Remove the plastic wrap and place the baking sheets, one at a time, in the center of the preheated oven, until the crackers are puffed and pale golden, about 12 minutes. Allow to cool on the baking sheets until firm. They will crisp as they cool.

The crackers can be stored in a sealed glass container at room temperature and should maintain their texture for at least 5 days. For longer storage, seal them tightly in a freezer-safe wrap or bag, and freeze for up to 2 months. Defrost at room temperature.

---

1 cup plus 2 tablespoons (156 g) all-purpose gluten-free flour (see page 2)

½ teaspoon baking soda

1 teaspoon baking powder

1 teaspoon (3 g) instant yeast

1 teaspoon (4 g) granulated sugar

½ teaspoon kosher salt, plus more for sprinkling

¼ teaspoon cream of tartar

2 tablespoons (24 g) nonhydrogenated vegetable shortening, at room temperature

3 tablespoons (42 g) unsalted butter, at room temperature

2 to 4 tablespoons seltzer, at room temperature

Nabisco Ritz Crackers, Original

MAKES ABOUT 25 CRACKERS

1 cup (140 g) all-purpose
gluten-free flour
(see page 2)

1½ teaspoons baking
powder

½ teaspoon (6 g)
granulated sugar

½ teaspoon smoked
Spanish paprika

¼ teaspoon kosher salt,
plus more for sprinkling

4 tablespoons (56)
unsalted butter, chopped
and chilled

1 tablespoon (14 g)
canola oil

¼ cup to ½ cup
(4 to 8 fluid ounces)
cold water

2 tablespoons (28 g)
unsalted butter, melted

*L*ight, buttery, and salty Ritz crackers are quite possibly the best cracker to pair with cheese. Imagine the surprise of your guests when they see gluten-free you munching on one of these with a nice slice of Gouda.

Preheat your oven to 375°F. Line rimmed baking sheets with parchment paper and set them aside.

In a large bowl, place the flour, baking powder, sugar, paprika, and ¼ teaspoon of kosher salt, and whisk to combine well. Using a pastry blender or two knives, cut the chopped, chilled butter into the flour mixture until it resembles small pebbles. Add the vegetable oil and stir to combine. Add ¼ cup of the water, stirring until the dough begins to come together. Add more water by the half-teaspoonful as necessary to bring the dough together. Transfer the dough to a piece of plastic wrap, and place in the refrigerator to chill for about 10 minutes.

Remove the dough from the refrigerator, place between two large sheets of unbleached parchment paper, and roll out until a bit more than ⅛ inch thick. Using a scalloped-edge 1¾-inch round cookie cutter, cut out shapes. Place about 1 inch apart from one another on the prepared baking sheets. With a toothpick, poke four to six holes in each cracker, toward the center to help them rise. Gather and reroll the scraps to cut out more crackers until you've used up the dough.

Place the baking sheets, one at a time, in the center of the preheated oven and bake until the crackers are just beginning to brown, about 7 minutes. Remove from the oven, brush the crackers with the melted butter, and sprinkle with salt. Allow to cool on the baking sheet. They will crisp as they cool.

The crackers can be stored in a sealed glass container at room temperature and should maintain their texture for at least 5 days. For longer storage, seal them tightly in a freezer-safe wrap or bag, and freeze for up to 2 months. Defrost at room temperature.

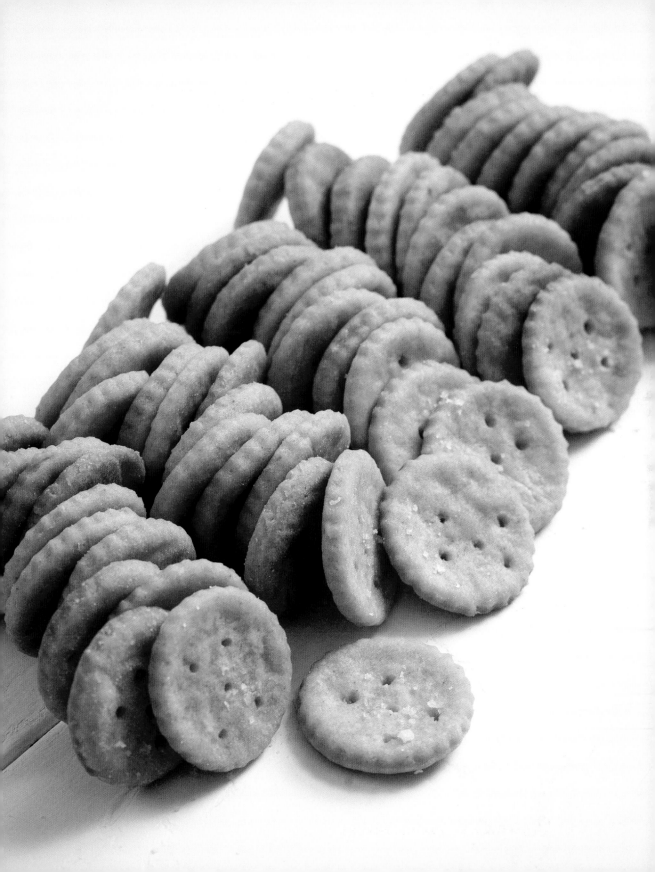

Nabisco Ritz Bits Cheese Sandwich Crackers

MAKES ABOUT 75 MINI CRACKER SANDWICHES

Crackers

1 cup (140 g) all-purpose gluten-free flour (see page 2)

1 ½ teaspoons baking powder

½ teaspoon (6 g) granulated sugar

½ teaspoon smoked Spanish paprika

¼ teaspoon kosher salt, plus more for sprinkling

4 tablespoons (56) unsalted butter, chopped and chilled

1 tablespoon (14 g) canola oil

¼ cup to ½ cup (4 to 8 fluid ounces) cold water

2 tablespoons (28 g) unsalted butter, melted

*I*f Ritz crackers are good, then it stands to reason that Ritz Bits Cheese Sandwich Crackers are better. They're mini, since that's how Nabisco makes them, but feel free to make them full size, like the Original crackers (page 188). Then fill and sandwich as directed.

Prepare the crackers: Preheat your oven to 375°F. Line rimmed baking sheets with unbleached parchment paper and set them aside.

In a large bowl, place the flour, baking powder, sugar, paprika, and ¼ teaspoon of salt, and whisk to combine well. Using a pastry blender or two knives, cut the chopped, chilled butter into the flour mixture until it resembles small pebbles. Add the vegetable oil and stir to combine. Add ¼ cup of the water, stirring until the dough begins to come together. Add more water by the half-teaspoonful as necessary to bring the dough together. Transfer the dough to a large piece of plastic wrap, and place in the refrigerator to chill for about 10 minutes.

Remove the dough from the refrigerator, place between two large sheets of unbleached parchment paper, and roll out until a bit more than ⅛ inch thick. Using a scalloped-edge ¾-inch round cookie cutter, cut out shapes. Place about 1 inch apart from one another on the prepared baking sheets. With a toothpick, poke two holes in each cracker, toward the center, to help them rise. Gather and reroll the scraps to cut out more crackers until you've used up the dough.

Place the baking sheets, one at a time, in the center of the preheated oven and bake until the crackers are just beginning to brown, about 7 minutes. Remove from the oven, brush the crackers with the melted butter, and sprinkle with salt. Allow to cool on the baking sheets. They will crisp as they cool.

While the crackers are cooling, prepare the filling: In a medium-size, heavy-bottomed saucepan, place the Cheddar cheese and evaporated milk. Cook, whisking frequently, over medium-high heat, until the cheese is completely melted. Add the flour, and whisk to combine well.

Continue to cook, stirring constantly, for another 2 minutes. Remove the saucepan from the heat, and stir in the butter until it is melted. The cheese will be somewhat thick, but still easily pourable. Transfer the cheese mixture to a medium-size heat-safe bowl, and allow to sit at room temperature until cool, about 10 minutes. Once the cheese mixture is cool, place it in a pastry bag fitted with a medium-size plain piping tip. Invert half of the cooled mini crackers. Pipe about ¼ teaspoon of cheese filling onto the inverted crackers. Top each with another cracker, right-side up, and press gently to form a sandwich.

These filled cracker sandwiches are best enjoyed the day that they are made. They can be stored in a sealed glass container at room temperature, but they will lose their texture within a couple of days due to the moisture in the filling. For longer storage, store the unfilled crackers themselves separately in a sealed glass container at room temperature for up to 5 days, or sealed tightly in a freezer-safe wrap or bag for up to 2 months and defrost at room temperature. Then, fill as directed before serving.

Cheese Filling

8 ounces Cheddar cheese, cut into a large dice

6 ounces (½ can) evaporated milk

1 tablespoon (9 g) all-purpose gluten-free flour (see page 2)

2 tablespoons (28 g) unsalted butter

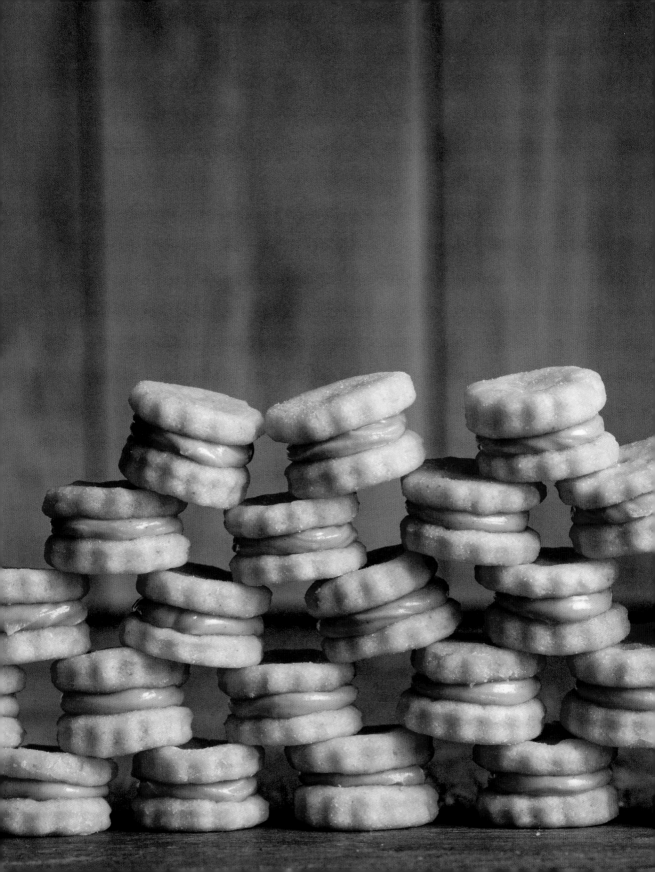

Nabisco Ritz Bits Peanut Butter Sandwich Crackers

MAKES ABOUT 75 MINI CRACKER SANDWICHES

*I*f you're looking for a stable mini peanut butter cracker sandwich, make the peanut butter filling just as directed. The mini cracker sandwiches are great for packing in school lunches (as long as your school isn't peanut-free, of course, in which case a no-stir almond butter, such as Barney Butter, would work as well). But if you're just making them to serve on a lazy Sunday, try using straight-up smooth, no-stir peanut butter as a filling. It'll get you snacking that much faster! Either way, you'll need a no-stir nut butter for a smooth filling that doesn't run.

Prepare the crackers: Preheat your oven to 375°F. Line rimmed baking sheets with unbleached parchment paper and set them aside.

In a large bowl, whisk well to combine the flour, baking powder, sugar, paprika, and ¼ teaspoon of salt, and whisk to combine well. Using a pastry blender or two knives, cut the chopped, chilled butter into the flour mixture until it resembles small pebbles. Add the vegetable oil and stir to combine. Add ¼ cup of the water, stirring until the dough begins to come together. Add more water by the half-teaspoonful as necessary to bring the dough together. Transfer the dough to a large piece of plastic wrap, and place in the refrigerator to chill for about 10 minutes.

Remove the dough from the refrigerator, place between two large sheets of unbleached parchment paper, and roll out until a bit more than ⅛ inch thick. Using a scalloped-edge ¾-inch round cookie cutter, cut out shapes. Place about 1 inch apart from one another on the prepared baking sheets. With a toothpick, poke two holes in each cracker, toward the center, to help them rise. Gather and reroll the scraps to cut out more crackers until you've used up the dough.

Place the baking sheets, one at a time, in the center of the preheated

Crackers

1 cup (140 g) all-purpose gluten-free flour (see page 2)

1½ teaspoons baking powder

½ teaspoon (6 g) granulated sugar

½ teaspoon smoked Spanish paprika

¼ teaspoon kosher salt, plus more for sprinkling

4 tablespoons (56) unsalted butter, chopped and chilled

1 tablespoon (14 g) canola oil

¼ cup to ½ cup (4 to 8 fluid ounces) cold water

2 tablespoons (28 g) unsalted butter, melted

Filling

Peanut Butter Filling (page 110)

oven and bake until the crackers are just beginning to brown, about 7 minutes. Remove from the oven, brush the crackers with the melted butter, and sprinkle with salt. Allow to cool on the baking sheets. They will crisp as they cool.

Prepare the Peanut Butter Filling. Place it in a pastry bag fitted with a medium-size plain piping tip. Invert half of the cooled mini crackers. Pipe about ¼ teaspoon of filling onto the inverted crackers. Top with another cracker, right-side up, and close gently to form a sandwich.

These filled cracker sandwiches are best enjoyed the day that they are made. They can be stored in a sealed glass container at room temperature, but they will lose their texture within a couple of days due to the moisture in the filling. For longer storage, store the unfilled crackers themselves separately in a sealed glass container at room temperature for up to 5 days, or sealed tightly in a freezer-safe wrap or bag for up to 2 months, and defrost at room temperature. Then, fill as directed before serving.

Nabisco Honey Maid Cinnamon Graham Crackers

MAKES ABOUT 20 GRAHAM CRACKERS

*T*hese cinnamon graham crackers have everything you'd expect—the lightly sweet taste, the crunchy texture, the waffling inside—all without using any actual graham flour. Just the right mix of granulated and brown sugar, with honey, molasses, and vanilla, plus a generous dusting of cinnamon sugar on the outside, bring the flavor all the way home. Cut them the right size and you could easily fool an unsuspecting four- or five-year-old. And isn't that at least half the fun of doing this—to fool people?

Prepare the crackers: Preheat your oven to 325°F. Line rimmed baking sheets with unbleached parchment paper and set them aside.

In a large bowl, place the flour, baking soda, baking powder, salt, cinnamon, and granulated sugar, and whisk to combine well. Add the brown sugar and whisk again, working out any lumps. Create a well in the center of the dry ingredients and add the shortening, honey, molasses, vanilla, egg, and 2 tablespoons of the milk, mixing to combine after each addition. Knead the dough together with your hands, adding more milk 1 teaspoonful at a time as necessary to help bring dough together.

Transfer the dough to a lightly floured piece of unbleached parchment paper and, sprinkling lightly with flour as necessary to prevent sticking, roll out the dough until it is about ¼ inch thick. Cut into 2 x 4-inch rectangles (or use a 2 x 4-inch rectangular cutter to cut out shapes) and place them about 1 inch apart from one another on the prepared baking sheets. Gather and reroll the scraps to cut out more crackers until you've used up the dough.

Prepare the topping: Combine the topping ingredients in a small bowl, and sprinkle the rectangles evenly with the cinnamon-sugar mixture.

Crackers

2 cups (280 g) all-purpose gluten-free flour (see page 2), plus more for sprinkling

¼ teaspoon baking soda

¼ teaspoon baking powder

⅛ teaspoon kosher salt

1 teaspoon ground cinnamon

¼ cup (50 g) granulated sugar

⅓ cup (72 g) packed light brown sugar

6 tablespoons (73 g) nonhydrogenated vegetable shortening, melted and cooled

2 tablespoons (42 g) honey

2 tablespoons (42 g) unsulfured molasses

½ teaspoon pure vanilla extract

CONTINUED ON PAGE 197

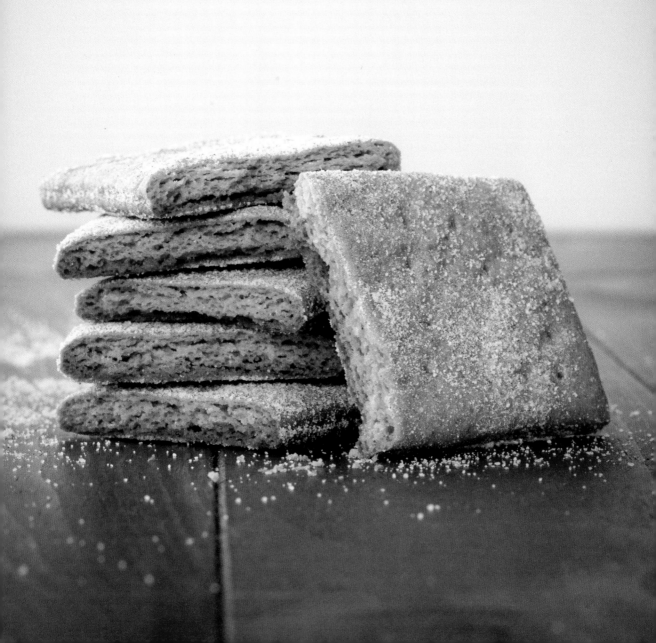

Place the baking sheets, one at a time, in the center of the preheated oven and bake until the crackers are golden brown all over and dry and firm to the touch, about 15 minutes. Remove from the oven and allow to cool completely on the baking sheets. They will crisp as they cool.

The crackers can be stored in a sealed glass container at room temperature and should maintain their texture for at least 5 days. For longer storage, seal them tightly in a freezer-safe wrap or bag, and freeze for up to 2 months. Defrost at room temperature.

CONTINUED FROM PAGE 195

1 egg (50 g, weighed out of shell), at room temperature, beaten

2 to 4 tablespoons milk, at room temperature

Topping

½ cup (100 g) granulated sugar

1½ teaspoons ground cinnamon

Nabisco Honey Maid Chocolate Graham Crackers

MAKES ABOUT 20 GRAHAM CRACKERS

1¾ cups (245 g) all-purpose gluten-free flour (see page 2), plus more for sprinkling

½ cup (40 g) unsweetened cocoa powder

¼ teaspoon baking soda

¼ teaspoon baking powder

⅛ teaspoon kosher salt

¼ cup (50 g) granulated sugar

⅓ cup (73 g) packed light brown sugar

5 tablespoons (60 g) nonhydrogenated vegetable shortening, melted and cooled

1 tablespoon (14 g) canola oil

2 tablespoons (42 g) honey

2 tablespoons (42 g) unsulfured molasses

*W*hen you make s'mores, consider making them with these chocolate graham crackers. Sandwich a marshmallow and a piece of chocolate between two chocolate graham crackers, and you've already taken s'mores to a new level, no extra effort required. The taste and texture are just as authentic as the cinnamon variety (see page 195). These are also perfect for crushing and using as a crust for a no-bake pie.

Preheat your oven to 325°F. Line rimmed baking sheets with unbleached parchment paper and set them aside.

In a large bowl, place the flour, cocoa powder, baking soda, baking powder, salt, and granulated sugar, and whisk to combine well. Add the brown sugar and whisk again, working out any lumps. Create a well in the center of the dry ingredients and add the shortening, honey, molasses, vanilla, egg, oil, and 2 tablespoons of the milk, mixing to combine after each addition. Knead the dough together with your hands, adding more milk 1 teaspoonful at a time as necessary to help bring the dough together.

Transfer the dough to a lightly floured piece of unbleached parchment paper and, sprinkling lightly with flour as necessary to prevent sticking, roll out the dough to about ¼ inch thick. Cut into 2 x 4-inch rectangles (or use a 2 x 4-inch rectangular cutter to cut out shapes) and place them about 1 inch apart from one another on the prepared baking sheets. Gather and reroll the scraps to cut out more crackers until you've used up the dough.

Place the baking sheets, one at a time, in the center of the preheated oven and bake until the crackers are dry and firm to the touch, about

15 minutes. Remove from the oven and allow to cool completely on the baking sheets. They will crisp as they cool.

The crackers can be stored in a sealed glass container at room temperature and should maintain their texture for at least 5 days. For longer storage, seal them tightly in a freezer-safe wrap or bag, and freeze for up to 2 months. Defrost at room temperature.

½ teaspoon pure vanilla extract

1 egg (50 g, weighed out of shell), at room temperature, beaten

2 to 4 tablespoons milk, at room temperature

Nabisco Barnum's Animal Crackers

MAKES ABOUT 60 COOKIES, DEPENDING UPON SIZE

1¼ cups (175 g) all-purpose gluten-free flour (see page 2), plus more for sprinkling

¼ cup (36 g) cornstarch

½ cup (58 g) confectioners' sugar

¼ teaspoon kosher salt

⅛ teaspoon baking soda

7 tablespoons (98 g) unsalted butter, at room temperature

1 egg (50 g, weighed out of shell), at room temperature, beaten

1 teaspoon pure vanilla extract

I've made animal cracker–shaped cookies before this recipe, but really, they just weren't authentic-tasting animal crackers. Until now. These animal crackers are buttery and light, and they melt in your mouth just like the kind in the little animal-decorated box. And just like the gluten-filled crackers in the box, they break relatively easily. If you're looking to make them just the same as I did in the photo, check the Resources section (see page 295) for the source of the best animal-shaped cutters.

Preheat your oven to 325°F. Line rimmed baking sheets with unbleached parchment paper and set them aside.

In a large bowl, place the flour, cornstarch, confectioners' sugar, salt, and baking soda, and whisk to combine well. Create a well in the center of the dry ingredients and add the butter, egg, and vanilla, mixing to combine after each addition. Knead the dough together with your hands.

Place the dough on a lightly floured surface, and roll it out a bit less than ¼ inch thick, sprinkling lightly with flour as necessary. Chill the dough in the refrigerator until firm, then cut out animal shapes and place them about 1 inch apart on the prepared baking sheets. Gather and reroll the scraps to cut out more crackers until you've used up the dough.

Place the baking sheets, one at a time, in the center of the preheated oven and bake until the crackers are just beginning to brown on edges, 8 to 10 minutes. Allow to cool completely on the baking sheets or they will break when you try to move them.

These can be stored in a sealed glass container at room temperature and should maintain their texture for at least 5 days. For longer storage, seal them tightly in a freezer-safe wrap or bag, and freeze for up to 2 months. Defrost at room temperature.

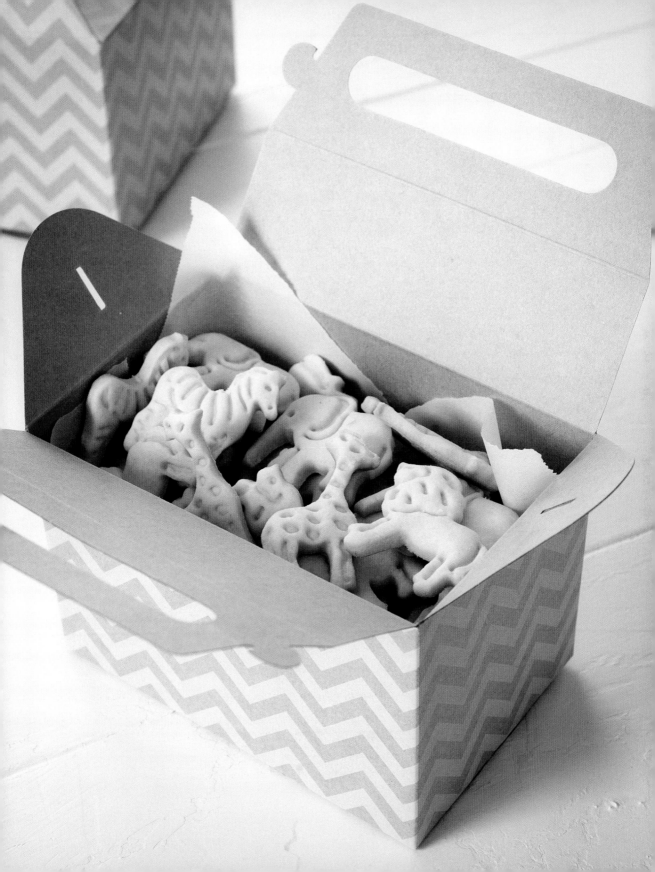

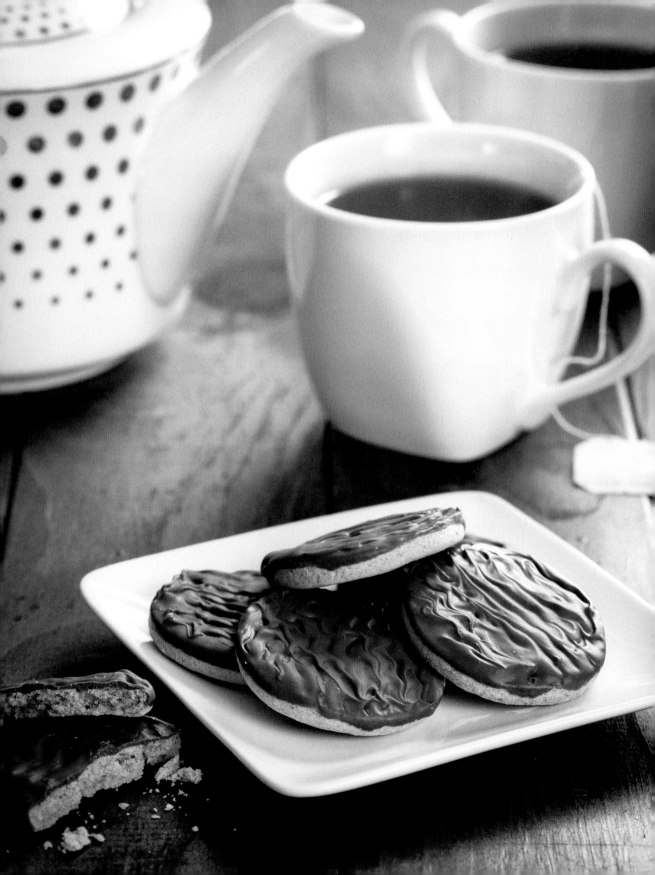

McVitie's Milk Chocolate Digestives

MAKES ABOUT 60 COOKIES

*T*hese digestive-style biscuits ended up in the crackers and crunchy snacks chapter for two reasons: First, they're British in origin and *biscuits* is what we Yanks call *cookies*. Second, they're really quite crunchy and very lightly sweet (only ½ cup of sugar in all sixty cookies) and taste more like crackers than out-and-out cookies to me. For the unfamiliar, digestives taste like a hearty cross between crackers and cookies, with a wheaty/whole-grain note. Here, they're dipped in chocolate, but they are delicious plain, too. To my British friends, pip-pip and cheerio!

Prepare the biscuits: Preheat your oven to 350°F. Line rimmed baking sheets with unbleached parchment paper and set them aside.

In a large bowl, place the gum-free flour blend, xanthan gum, cornstarch, whole-grain flour blend, nonfat dry milk, and salt, and whisk to combine well. Add the brown sugar and whisk again, working out any lumps. Create a well in the center of the dry ingredients and add the butter, Lyle's golden syrup, and milk, mixing to combine after each addition. The dough will be thick and sticky.

Place the dough on a lightly floured surface and, sprinkling with flour as necessary to prevent sticking, roll it out about ⅜ inch thick. Cut out shapes with a floured 2-inch round cookie cutter. If the rounds are too sticky to handle, place the rolled-out dough in the freezer until firm, about 10 minutes. Place the cut-out rounds of dough about 1 inch apart from one another on the prepared baking sheets, and prick randomly all over the surface of each round with a toothpick or wooden skewer. Gather and reroll the scraps to cut out more crackers until you've used up the dough.

Place the baking sheets, one at a time, in the center of the preheated oven and bake until the biscuits are lightly golden brown on the edges and dry to the touch, about 10 minutes. Remove from the oven and allow

---

Biscuits

1¼ cups (175 g) basic gum-free gluten-free flour blend (see page 7), plus more for sprinkling

¼ teaspoon xanthan gum

¼ cup (36 g) cornstarch

1¼ cups (175 g) whole-grain gluten-free flour blend (see page 8)

3 tablespoons plus 1 teaspoon (20 g) nonfat dry milk, ground into a finer powder

¼ teaspoon kosher salt

½ cup (109 g) packed light brown sugar

8 tablespoons (112 g) unsalted butter, at room temperature

2 tablespoons (42 g) Lyle's golden syrup

½ cup (4 fluid ounces) milk, at room temperature

CONTINUED ON PAGE 204

CONTINUED FROM PAGE 203

Chocolate Glaze

12 ounces milk chocolate, chopped

3 tablespoons (42 g) virgin coconut oil

to cool on the baking sheets for 10 minutes before transferring to a wire rack to cool completely.

While the biscuits are cooling, prepare the glaze: Line a rimmed baking sheet with parchment or waxed paper, and set it just to the side. In a medium-size, heat-safe bowl, place the chocolate and coconut oil and melt according to the instructions on page 21. Allow to cool slightly to until the mixture begins to thicken. Dip the bottoms of all the cookies in the chocolate, and place chocolate side up on a piece of parchment or waxed paper. Before the chocolate has a chance to set, drag the tines of a fork in a wiggly pattern through the melted chocolate coating. Allow the cookies to sit until the chocolate is set.

These are best enjoyed the day they are finished by being dipped in chocolate. The finished cookies can be stored in a sealed glass container at room temperature for about 2 days. For longer storage, seal the finished cookies tightly in a freezer-safe wrap or bag, and freeze for up to 2 months. Defrost at room temperature. The chocolate coating may bloom a bit over time, but it won't affect the taste at all.

Snyder's of Hanover Pretzel Rods

MAKES ABOUT 25 PRETZELS

*T*hese are the long, thin, crunchy pretzel rods we miss. Luckily for us, Snyder's does make a few varieties of gluten-free pretzels, and they actually taste quite good. But the company's gluten-free pretzels cost nearly three times as much as its regular pretzels—and Snyder's doesn't make gluten-free pretzel rods. I've made these crunchy pretzel rods with the lovely yeasted dough from the Pretzel Rolls on page 153 of *Gluten-Free on a Shoestring Bakes Bread* (reprinted below). As is traditional with homemade pretzels, after shaping and rising, these are first boiled in a simple baking soda bath before being baked. This step is crucial, as it both helps the pretzels to brown in the oven and prevents them from rising too much during baking. These take a bit of time, but once you dip the first crispy, crunchy, and salty homemade pretzel rod in a bit of mustard, you'll be so glad you went for it.

Place the bread flour, dry milk, yeast, cream of tartar, and brown sugar in the bowl of a stand mixer, and use a handheld whisk to combine well. Add the salt, and whisk to combine. Add the butter and water, and mix on low speed with the dough hook until combined. If you don't have a stand mixer, you can use a 5-speed hand mixer with dough hook attachments. Raise the mixer speed to medium and knead for about 5 minutes. The dough will be quite sticky, but it should be smooth and stretchy. Spray a silicone spatula lightly with cooking oil spray, and scrape down the sides of the bowl.

Transfer the dough to a lightly oiled bowl or proofing bucket large enough for it to rise to double its size, and cover with an oiled piece of plastic wrap or the oiled top to your proofing bucket. Be sure that your refrigerator does not run too cold (mine is set to 32°F) or the yeast will not be active, and that the proofing container you use is well sealed or

---

3¼ cups (455 g) gluten-free bread flour (see page 8), plus more for sprinkling

7 tablespoons (42 g) nonfat dry milk, ground into a finer powder

2 teaspoons (6 g) instant yeast

¼ teaspoon cream of tartar

1 tablespoon (14 g) packed light brown sugar

1 teaspoon kosher salt

4 tablespoons (56 g) unsalted butter, at room temperature

1¼ cups plus 2 tablespoons (1 fluid ounce) warm water (about 95°F)

Baking soda bath, for boiling (6 cups water plus 1 tablespoon baking soda and 1 teaspoon kosher salt)

Coarse salt, for sprinkling

---

the dough will dry out and will not rise. Place the dough in the refrigerator for at least 12 hours and up to 4 days. If you don't want to wait for the dough to rise slowly in the refrigerator, which allows both for flavor development and for the dough to become much easier to handle, you can place the covered dough in a warm, draft-free location to rise until doubled in size. Then, place it, still covered tightly, in the refrigerator to chill for at least 30 minutes and continue with the rest of the recipe.

On baking day, line two rimmed baking sheets with unbleached parchment paper, grease them lightly with cooking oil spray, and set them aside. Remove the dough from the refrigerator and turn it out onto a lightly floured surface. Knead the dough until smoother in the following manner: With the help of an oiled bench scraper, keep moving the dough as you shape it, particularly if it begins to stick to the surface or your hands. Scrape the dough off the floured surface with the bench scraper, then fold the dough over itself. Sprinkle the dough very lightly with flour, scrape the dough up again, and fold it over itself again. Repeat scraping and folding in this manner until the dough has become smoother. Keep the outside of the dough and the surface covered in a light coating of flour as you shape it. Handle the dough with a *very light touch* to avoid kneading the flour into the dough, which might dry it out and result in a tight, unpleasant crumb. Remember to use a very light touch, sprinkle only very lightly with additional bread flour, and always work with cold dough as it is much easier to shape.

With a floured bench scraper, divide the dough in half. Cover one piece of dough loosely with a clean towel to prevent it from drying out. Working with the other half, divide it into four equal pieces. Roll each piece of dough (pressing down and out with your palms) into a rope about 10 inches long. Using a floured bench scraper or sharp knife, slice each rope in half. Place each piece of shaped dough 2 inches apart from one another on the prepared baking sheets. Repeat the process with the other half of dough. Dust all the shaped pieces of dough lightly with flour, then cover with lightly oiled plastic wrap. Set in a warm, draft-free location to rise until nearly doubled in size, about 40 minutes. The sticks will swell in every direction as they rise, but the doubling will not be as obvious as it is with a larger piece of dough.

As the dough nears the end of its rise, preheat your oven to 325°F. In a large pot, make the baking soda bath by dissolving the baking soda and salt in about 6 cups of water, and bringing it to a rolling boil over medium-high heat. Once the dough has finished rising, place the risen

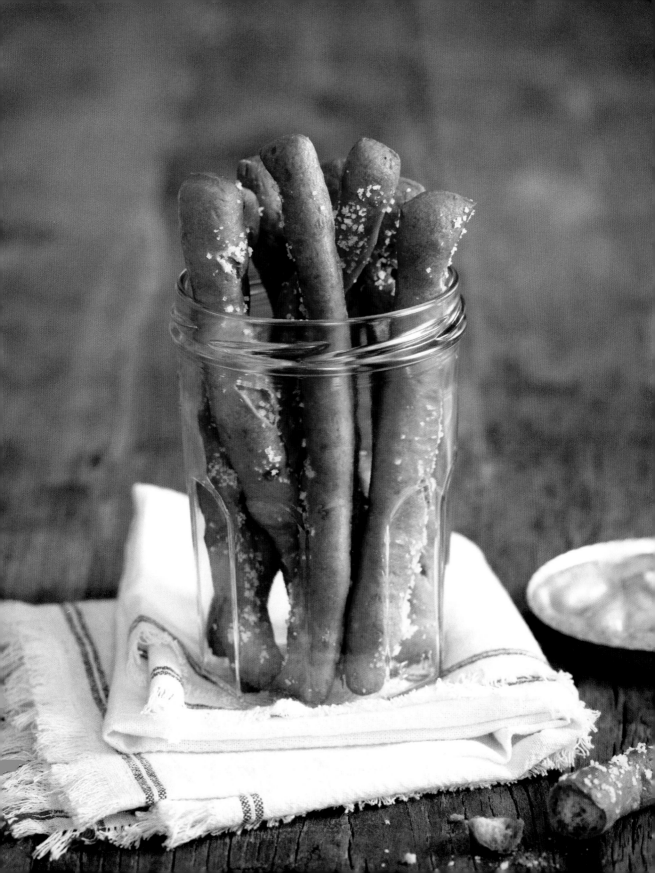

sticks a few at a time in the boiling baking soda bath for about 30 seconds per side. Remove the boiled dough with a strainer and return the pieces to the baking sheet, about 1½ inches apart from one another. Using a very sharp knife, slash each piece of dough at a 45-degree angle in two or three places, about ¼ inch deep. Sprinkle generously with coarse salt.

Place the baking sheets in the center of the preheated oven. Bake until the pretzel rods are a deep golden brown all over and crisp, 40 to 55 minutes. Remove from the oven and allow to cool briefly. They will continue to crisp as they cool.

The pretzels can be stored in a sealed glass container at room temperature and should maintain their texture for at least 5 days. For longer storage, seal them tightly in a freezer-safe wrap or bag, and freeze for up to 2 months. Defrost at room temperature.

CHAPTER 5

Breakfast & Fruity Treats

From Grab-and-Go Breakfast Bars to Fruit-Filled Goodies

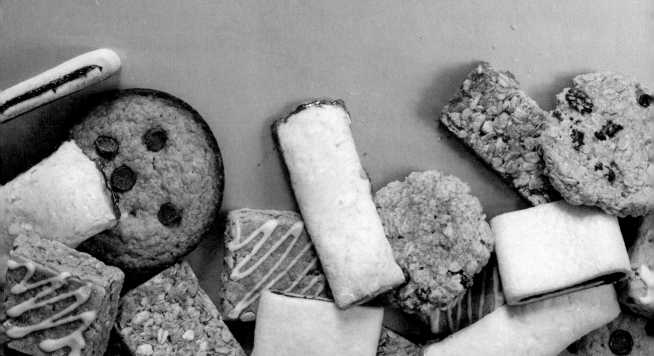

Quaker Oatmeal to Go, Brown Sugar Cinnamon

MAKES 16 BARS

Squares

2 cups (280 g) all-purpose gluten-free flour (see page 2)

1 cup (120 g) certified gluten-free oat flour

2 tablespoons (15 g) certified gluten-free oat bran

¼ teaspoon baking soda

½ teaspoon baking powder

½ teaspoon kosher salt

1 teaspoon ground cinnamon

1 cup (218 g) packed light brown sugar

¾ cup (75 g) certified gluten-free old-fashioned rolled oats

8 tablespoons (112 g) unsalted butter, melted and cooled

2 eggs (100 g, weighed out of shell), at room temperature, beaten

CONTINUED ON PAGE 212

These bars have whole grains in the form of oat flour, oat bran, and old-fashioned rolled oats, but I'm not entirely convinced that they're a completely healthy breakfast. If you make them as directed below, they will taste just like the original: chewy and sweet squares that really do taste like you're holding brown sugar and cinnamon oatmeal in your hand, rather than enjoying it by the spoonful. If you'd like to make them a bit more virtuous, try swapping out the butter for virgin coconut oil and the brown sugar for an equal amount, by weight, of coconut palm sugar. And I guess, regretfully, skip the glaze. They won't taste like the original, though, so promise you'll treat yourself to the true clone recipe at least once before you go tinkering?

First, prepare the squares: Preheat your oven to 325°F. Line a rimmed baking sheet with unbleached parchment paper and set it aside.

In a large bowl, place the flour, oat flour, oat bran, baking soda, baking powder, salt, and cinnamon, and whisk to combine well. Add the brown sugar and rolled oats, and mix to combine, working out any lumps. Create a well in the center of the dry ingredients and add the butter, eggs, vanilla, and molasses, and mix until the dough comes together. It will be thick and very moist.

Place the dough between two sheets of unbleached parchment paper and pat and roll out into an 8-inch square that is about ¾ inch thick. Remove the top sheet of parchment paper and, using a bench scraper or large, sharp knife, slice into sixteen 2-inch squares. Place the squares about 1 inch apart on the prepared baking sheet, and place in the refrigerator to chill until firm, about 10 minutes. Remove the pan from the refrigerator, place in the center of the preheated oven, and bake, rotating once during baking, until the bars are mostly firm to the touch and just beginning to brown lightly on top, 12 to 14 minutes. Remove from the oven and allow to cool completely on the pan.

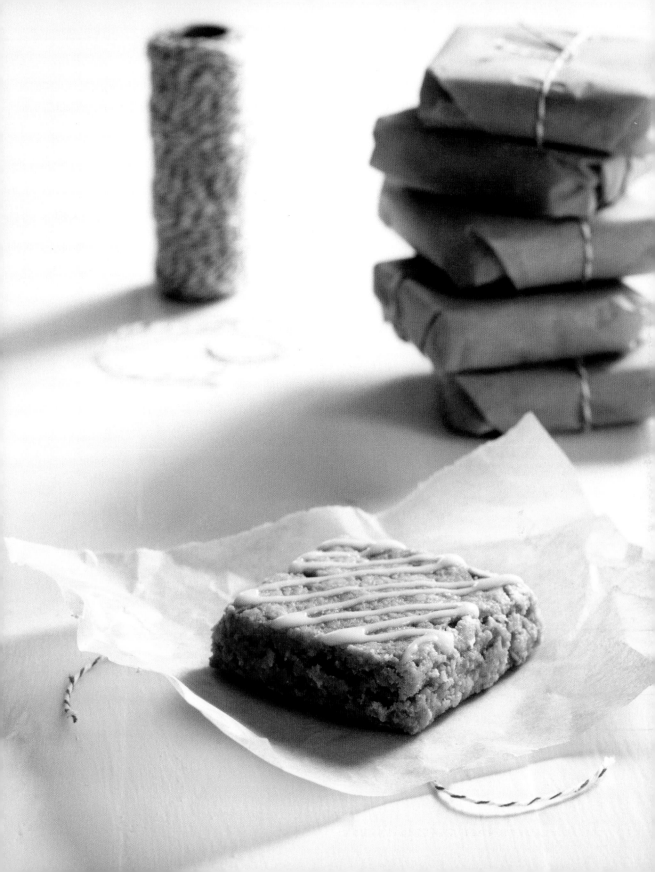

CONTINUED FROM PAGE 210

2 teaspoons pure vanilla extract

2 tablespoons (42 g) unsulfured molasses

Glaze

1 cup (115 g) confectioners' sugar

⅛ teaspoon table salt

1 to 2 tablespoons (½ to 1 fluid ounce) milk, at room temperature

1 tablespoon (14 g) unsalted butter, at room temperature

½ teaspoon pure vanilla extract

While the squares are cooling, prepare the glaze: In a medium-size bowl, place the confectioners' sugar and salt and whisk to combine well. Add 1 tablespoon of the milk and the butter and vanilla, and mix until a thick, smooth paste forms. If the paste is too thick to pipe, add more milk by the half-teaspoonful until you reach the proper consistency. Once the squares have cooled completely, pipe a zigzag pattern of glaze on top of each square. Allow to set at room temperature.

These can be stored in a sealed glass or plastic container at room temperature and should maintain their texture for about 5 days. For longer storage, wrap individually in freezer-safe wrap, and freeze for up to 2 months. Defrost at room temperature.

Quaker Breakfast Cookies, Oatmeal Chocolate Chip

MAKES 14 COOKIES

Breakfast cookies should be just as these are: soft, tender, and thick. There are only 3 ounces of miniature chocolate chips in the whole batch of fourteen large cookies, enough to give you the taste of chocolate in each cookie but not so much that it doesn't taste like breakfast. The same sugar substitutions can be made here as in the oatmeal raisin version on page 214. This chocolate chip variety is also sweetened with a bit of brown sugar, which can be replaced with an equal amount by weight of coconut palm sugar.

Preheat your oven to 350°F. Line a rimmed baking sheet with unbleached parchment paper and set it aside.

In a large bowl, place the oat flour, all-purpose flour, baking soda, and salt, and whisk to combine well. Add the oats and brown sugar and mix to combine, working out any lumps. Create a well in the center of the dry ingredients, and add the shortening, corn syrup, golden syrup, eggs, and applesauce, mixing to combine after each addition. Add the cornstarch-dusted chocolate chips, and mix until evenly distributed throughout. The dough will be thick and sticky. Drop pieces of dough, about 2 tablespoonsful each, about 2 inches apart from one another on the prepared baking sheet. With wet fingers, spread each into a disk about ¼ inch thick.

Place the baking sheet in the center of the preheated oven and bake until the cookies are beginning to brown around the edges and set in the center, about 12 minutes. Remove from the oven and allow to cool on the baking sheet for 10 minutes, or until firm, before transferring to a wire rack to cool completely.

These can be stored in a sealed glass or plastic container at room temperature and should maintain their texture for about 5 days. For longer storage, wrap individually in freezer-safe wrap, and freeze for up to 2 months. Defrost at room temperature.

1 cup (120 g) certified gluten-free oat flour

½ cup (70 g) all-purpose gluten-free flour (see page 2)

½ teaspoon baking soda

¼ teaspoon kosher salt

1¼ cups (125 g) certified gluten-free old-fashioned rolled oats

2 tablespoons (27 g) packed light brown sugar

5 tablespoons (60 g) nonhydrogenated vegetable shortening, melted and cooled

4 tablespoons (84 g) light corn syrup

4 tablespoons (84 g) Lyle's golden syrup

2 eggs (100 g, weighed out of shell), at room temperature, beaten

½ cup (120 g) smooth unsweetened applesauce

3 ounces miniature chocolate chips, tossed with 1 teaspoon cornstarch

Quaker Breakfast Cookies, Oatmeal Raisin

MAKES 14 COOKIES

1 cup (120 g) certified gluten-free oat flour

½ cup (70 g) all-purpose gluten-free flour (see page 2)

½ teaspoon baking soda

¼ teaspoon kosher salt

1 teaspoon ground cinnamon

1¼ cups (125 g) certified gluten-free old-fashioned rolled oats

5 tablespoons (60 g) nonhydrogenated vegetable shortening, melted and cooled

4 tablespoons (84 g) light corn syrup

4 tablespoons (84 g) Lyle's golden syrup

2 eggs (100 g, weighed out of shell), at room temperature, beaten

½ cup (120 g) smooth unsweetened applesauce

3 ounces raisins, tossed with 1 teaspoon cornstarch

These generously sized cinnamon-kissed oatmeal raisin breakfast cookies are super moist and tender, which isn't a given when applesauce takes the place of a fair amount of the fat in a recipe. If you'd like to cut back on the sugar, try replacing half of the total liquid sugars (the light corn syrup and Lyle's golden syrup) with an equal amount, by weight, of Swerve (see page 16). Just add another tablespoon of applesauce to make up for the lost liquid. If you can't find Lyle's golden syrup, try replacing it with honey (see page 12 for a more complete discussion of ingredients and substitutions).

Preheat your oven to 350°F. Line a rimmed baking sheet with unbleached parchment paper and set it aside.

In a large bowl, place the oat flour, all-purpose flour, baking soda, salt, and cinnamon, and whisk to combine well. Add the oats and mix to combine. Create a well in the center of the dry ingredients, and add the shortening, corn syrup, golden syrup, eggs, and applesauce, mixing to combine after each addition. Add the cornstarch-dusted raisins, and mix until evenly distributed throughout. The dough will be thick and sticky. Drop pieces of dough, about 2 tablespoonsful each, about 2 inches apart from one another on the prepared baking sheet. With wet fingers, spread each into a disk about ¼ inch thick.

Place in the center of the preheated oven and bake until the cookies are beginning to brown around the edges and set in the center, about 12 minutes. Remove from the oven and allow to cool on the baking sheet for 10 minutes, or until firm, before transferring to a wire rack to cool completely.

These can be stored in a sealed glass or plastic container at room temperature and should maintain their texture for about 5 days. For longer storage, wrap individually in freezer-safe wrap, and freeze for up to 2 months. Defrost at room temperature.

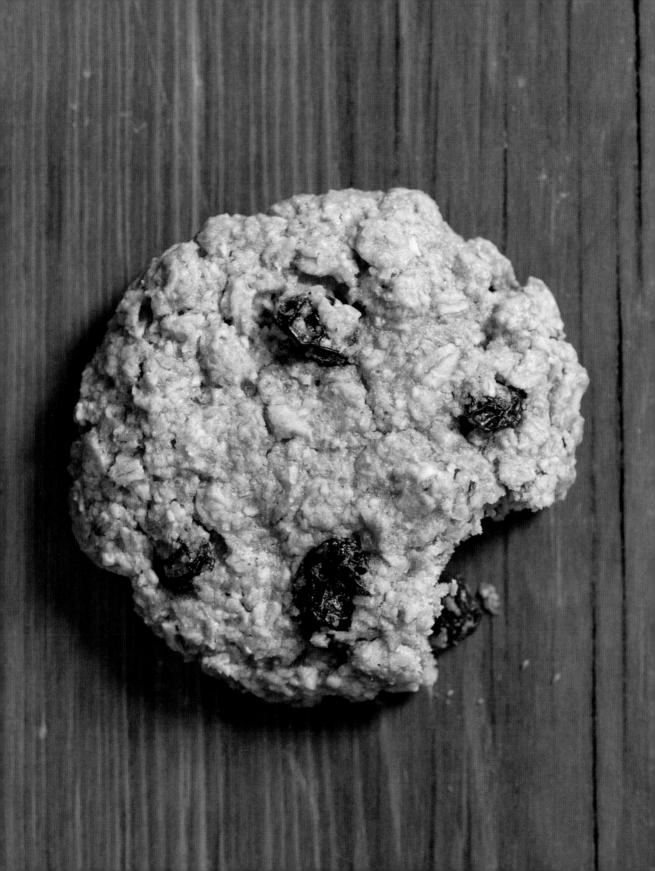

Quaker Instant Oatmeal, Cinnamon & Spice

MAKES 8 SERVINGS

3 cups (330 g) certified gluten-free quick-cooking oats

2 cups (240 g) certified gluten-free oat flour

½ cup (48 g) nonfat dry milk, ground into a finer powder

⅛ teaspoon kosher salt

1 teaspoon ground cinnamon

¼ teaspoon freshly ground nutmeg

¾ cup (164 g) packed light brown sugar

I generally make it a policy to buy only one type of certified gluten-free oats: old-fashioned whole oats. With all the types of flours and other baking ingredients I have to keep in stock in my pantry, I can't justify stocking quick-cooking oats or oat flour. The difference between the various forms of oats is generally one of grind, so I just process old-fashioned rolled oats for either quick-cooking oats or oat flour: pulse three or four times in a food processor for the former, and continuously until I have a fine powder for the latter. Combining quick-cooking oats and oat flour in this instant oatmeal is a great way to help the mixture come together without having to add too much liquid. Dividing the mixture into pre-measured individual portions, just like the packaged product, makes for quick and easy mornings.

Place all the ingredients in a large bowl and whisk to combine well. Divide into eight servings, each about ¾ cup, and place each in a separate sealed container or resealable plastic bag for later use. They will keep until the expiration date on your nonfat dry milk, the most perishable ingredient.

When ready to use, pour each portion into a separate heat-safe bowl or cup and add ¼ to ⅓ cup of hot (but not boiling) water to achieve the desired consistency. Serve immediately.

Quaker Instant Oatmeal, Strawberries & Cream

MAKES 8 SERVINGS

*A*dding freeze-dried strawberries to this instant oatmeal variety gives it a great big flavor boost without adding extra sugar. Just Tomatoes, Etc.! brand makes every imaginable freeze-dried fruit and vegetable under the sun and sells them in many major grocery stores. I also buy freeze-dried fruit from Nuts.com, which even sells it in already powdered form.

Place all the ingredients in a large bowl and whisk to combine well. Divide into eight servings, each about ¾ cup, and place each in a separate sealed container or resealable plastic bag for later use. They will keep until the expiration date on your nonfat dry milk, the most perishable ingredient.

    When ready to use, pour into a heat-safe bowl or cup and add ¼ to ⅓ cup of hot (but not boiling) water to achieve desired consistency. Serve immediately.

---

3 cups (330 g) certified gluten-free quick-cooking oats (see headnote on page 216 for details)

2 cups (240 g) certified gluten-free oat flour

½ cup (48 g) nonfat dry milk, ground into a finer powder

⅛ teaspoon kosher salt

2 cups (56 g) freeze-dried strawberries, ground into a fine powder

¾ cup (164 g) packed light brown sugar

Kellogg's Nutri-Grain Cereal Bars, Apple Cinnamon

MAKES 15 BARS

Bar Dough

2 cups (280 g) all-purpose gluten-free flour (see page 2), plus more for sprinkling

¼ cup (36 g) cornstarch

6 tablespoons (36 g) nonfat dry milk, ground into a finer powder

1 cup (120 g) certified gluten-free oat flour

¼ teaspoon baking soda

½ teaspoon baking powder

½ teaspoon kosher salt

¾ cup (75 g) certified gluten-free old-fashioned rolled oats

¾ cup (150 g) granulated sugar

½ cup (114 g) plain yogurt, at room temperature

2 tablespoons (28 g) canola oil

2 teaspoons pure vanilla extract

The texture of these cereal bars is just like the original, but in some ways they're even better. If you recall, the original bars tend to fall apart rather easily once they're unwrapped. These bars hold their shape even better, and the smooth, sweet apple cinnamon filling and whole grains make them a family favorite. The plain yogurt can be replaced with an equal amount by weight of sour cream (just not nonfat).

Prepare the bar dough: Preheat your oven to 350°F. Line rimmed baking sheets with unbleached parchment paper and set them aside.

In a large bowl, place the flour, cornstarch, nonfat dry milk, oat flour, baking soda, baking powder, and salt, and whisk to combine well. Add the oats and sugar, and mix to combine well. Create a well in the center of the dry ingredients, and add the yogurt, canola oil, vanilla, egg, and water, mixing to combine after each addition. Knead the dough together with your hands, adding more water as necessary until the dough holds together. It will be sticky and somewhat stiff. Transfer the dough to a lightly floured surface and roll the dough out into a rectangle about ¼ inch thick (no thinner or the filling will leak during baking). Using a sharp knife or pizza or pastry wheel, cut the dough into 4-inch squares, gathering and rerolling scraps as necessary. Dust the pieces of dough lightly with flour and place them in a stack. Place the dough in the refrigerator to chill while you make the filling.

Prepare the filling: Place all the filling ingredients in a small saucepan, mix to combine well, and cook over medium-low heat, stirring frequently, until reduced and thickened, about 4 minutes. Allow to cool briefly.

Once the filling has cooled, place about 2 tablespoons of it down the center third of each square of dough, and fold the ends over each other to cover the filling. Pinch the ends of each bar together to seal. If the dough is too cold from being in the refrigerator, it will crack during folding. If it begins to crack, allow it to sit at room temperature until it becomes more pliable before continuing to shape the bars. Place the bars about 2 inches apart from one another on the prepared baking sheets.

Place the baking sheets, one at a time, in the center of the preheated oven and bake until the bars are very lightly golden brown all over, and slightly darker on the edges, about 15 minutes. Allow to cool until firm on the baking sheets before transferring to a wire rack to cool completely.

The baked bars can be stored in a sealed glass container at room temperature and should maintain their texture for at least 3 days. For longer storage, wrap individually in freezer-safe wrap, and freeze for up to 2 months. Defrost at room temperature.

1 egg (50 g, weighed out of shell), at room temperature, beaten

¼ cup (2 ounces) lukewarm water, plus more as necessary

Apple Cinnamon Filling

1 cup (240 g) smooth unsweetened applesauce

1 teaspoon (3 g) cornstarch

1 teaspoon ground cinnamon

———————

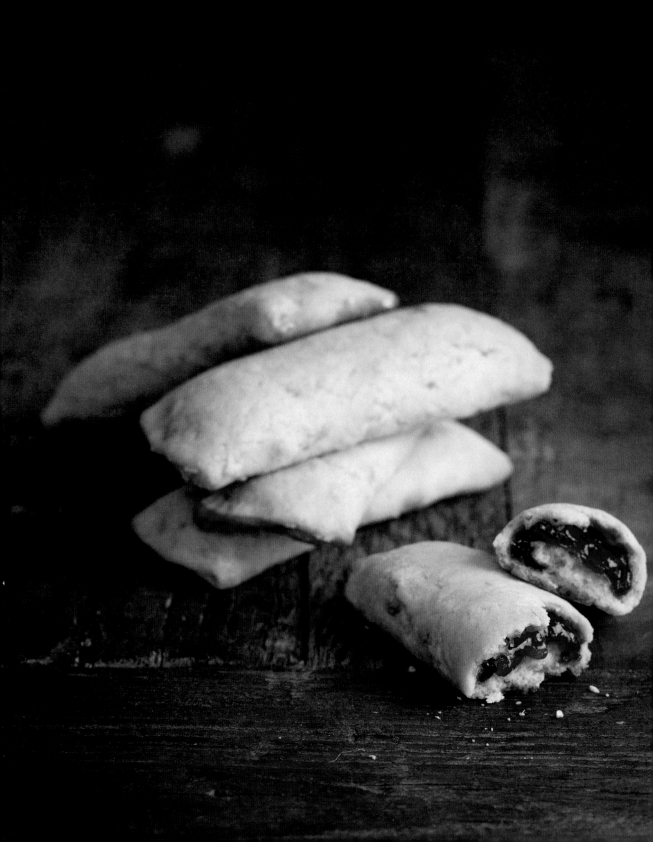

Kellogg's Nutri-Grain Cereal Bars, Strawberry

MAKES 15 BARS

Sweeter than their apple cinnamon cousins, these cereal bars taste a bit more like a treat. Be sure to find seedless strawberry preserves or jam, as the only real chewy texture should come from the old-fashioned rolled oats, not from strawberry seeds. Polaner makes really nice seedless strawberry preserves.

Prepare the bar dough: Preheat your oven to 350°F. Line rimmed baking sheets with unbleached parchment paper and set them aside.

To make the dough, in a large bowl, place the flour, cornstarch, nonfat dry milk, oat flour, baking soda, baking powder, and salt, and whisk to combine well. Add the oats and sugar, and mix to combine well. Create a well in the center of the dry ingredients, and add the yogurt, canola oil, vanilla, egg, and water, mixing to combine after each addition. Knead the dough together with your hands, adding more water as necessary until the dough holds together. It will be sticky and somewhat stiff. Transfer the dough to a lightly floured surface and roll the dough out into a rectangle about ¼ inch thick (no thinner or the filling will leak during baking). Using a sharp knife or pizza or pastry wheel, cut the dough into 4-inch squares, gathering and rerolling scraps as necessary. Dust the pieces of dough lightly with flour and place them in a stack. Place the dough in the refrigerator to chill for about 5 minutes to make it easier to handle. Be careful not to chill the dough for too long or it will crack during folding. If it begins to crack as you shape the bars, allow it to sit at room temperature until it becomes more pliable before continuing to shape the bars.

To shape the bars, place about 2 tablespoons of strawberry preserves down the center third of each square of dough, and fold the ends over each other to cover the filling. Pinch the ends of each bar together to seal. Place the bars about 2 inches apart from one another on the prepared baking sheets.

Bar Dough

2 cups (280 g) all-purpose gluten-free flour (see page 2), plus more for sprinkling

¼ cup (36 g) cornstarch

6 tablespoons (36 g) nonfat dry milk, ground into a finer powder

1 cup (120 g) certified gluten-free oat flour

¼ teaspoon baking soda

½ teaspoon baking powder

½ teaspoon kosher salt

¾ cup (75 g) certified gluten-free old-fashioned rolled oats

¾ cup (150 g) granulated sugar

½ cup (114 g) plain yogurt (or sour cream), at room temperature

2 tablespoons (28 g) canola oil

CONTINUED ON PAGE 222

CONTINUED FROM PAGE 221

2 teaspoons pure vanilla extract

1 egg (50 g, weighed out of shell), at room temperature, beaten

¼ cup (2 ounces) lukewarm water, plus more as necessary

Filling

6 ounces seedless strawberry preserves

Place the baking sheets, one at a time, in the center of the preheated oven and bake until the bars are very lightly golden brown all over and slightly darker on the edges, about 15 minutes. Allow to cool until firm on the baking sheets before transferring to a wire rack to cool completely.

The finished bars can be stored in a sealed glass container at room temperature and should maintain their texture for at least 3 days. For longer storage, wrap individually in freezer-safe wrap, and freeze for up to 2 months. Defrost at room temperature.

Kellogg's Frosted Strawberry Pop-Tarts Toaster Pastries

MAKES 12 PASTRIES

*A*s a child of the 1980s, I ate Pop-Tarts for breakfast every single morning before school. At first, I thought that they *had* to be toasted. They're called toaster pastries, after all. The day that I discovered that they were still quite delicious right out of the package was the day I could sleep about five minutes later every school morning. I like these frosted pastries best when they aren't toasted: light, tender, and delicious! But of course you can toast them, if you like.

Prepare the crust: Preheat your oven to 350°F. Line a large rimmed baking sheet with unbleached parchment paper and set it aside.

In a large bowl, place the flour, cornstarch, salt, and sugar, and whisk to combine well. Create a well in the center of the dry ingredients, and add the butter, vanilla, egg, and 2 fluid ounces of the milk, mixing to combine after each addition. The dough will be thick. Knead the dough with your hands until it is smooth, adding more milk by the half-teaspoonful as necessary to bring the dough together. Place the dough on a lightly floured surface and dust lightly with flour to prevent the dough from sticking to the rolling pin. Roll out the dough ¼ inch thick and slice it into 3½ x 4½-inch rectangles. Gather and reroll any scraps, and cut out as many more rectangles as possible (it should be at least twenty-four rectangles). If the dough becomes difficult to handle at any point, wrap it in plastic wrap and place it in the freezer to chill briefly.

Place 1 tablespoon of strawberry jelly on the center of half of the rectangles of dough, and spread into an even layer, leaving a ¾-inch border clean on all sides of the rectangle. Cover with the remaining rectangles of dough and press all around the clean edge to seal. Using a sharp knife or pastry or pizza wheel, cut off about ½ inch of dough around all sides of each pastry. Place the pastries about 2 inches apart

Crust

2¼ cups (315 g) all-purpose gluten-free flour (see page 2), plus more for sprinkling

¼ cup (36 g) cornstarch

¼ teaspoon kosher salt

¾ cup (150 g) granulated sugar

8 tablespoons (112 g) unsalted butter, melted and cooled

1 teaspoon pure vanilla extract

1 egg (50 g weighed out of shell), at room temperature, beaten

4 to 6 tablespoons (2 to 3 fluid ounces) milk, at room temperature

Filling

¾ cup seedless strawberry jelly or jam

CONTINUED ON PAGE 224

CONTINUED FROM PAGE 223

Glaze

2 cups (230 g) confectioners' sugar

1 tablespoon (½ fluid ounce) lukewarm water, plus more by the half-teaspoonful

Multicolored gluten-free nonpareils, for sprinkling

from one another on the prepared baking sheet. Dock the pastries by piercing randomly on top with a toothpick or wooden skewer. Place the baking sheet in the center of the preheated oven and bake until the pastries are very lightly golden brown around the edges and just set in the center, about 8 minutes.

Remove from the oven and allow to cool on the baking sheet for 10 minutes before transferring to a wire rack to cool completely.

While the pastries are cooling, prepare the glaze: In a medium-size bowl, place the confectioners' sugar and 1 tablespoon of the water, and mix until combined into a thick paste. Add more water by the half-teaspoonful as necessary to create a thickly pourable glaze. Spread the glaze thickly on top of each cooled pastry and sprinkle lightly with nonpareils. Allow to set at room temperature before serving.

The finished pastries can be stored in a sealed glass container at room temperature and should maintain their texture for at least 3 days. For longer storage, wrap individually in freezer-safe wrap, and freeze for up to 2 months. Defrost at room temperature or unwrap and defrost in the toaster.

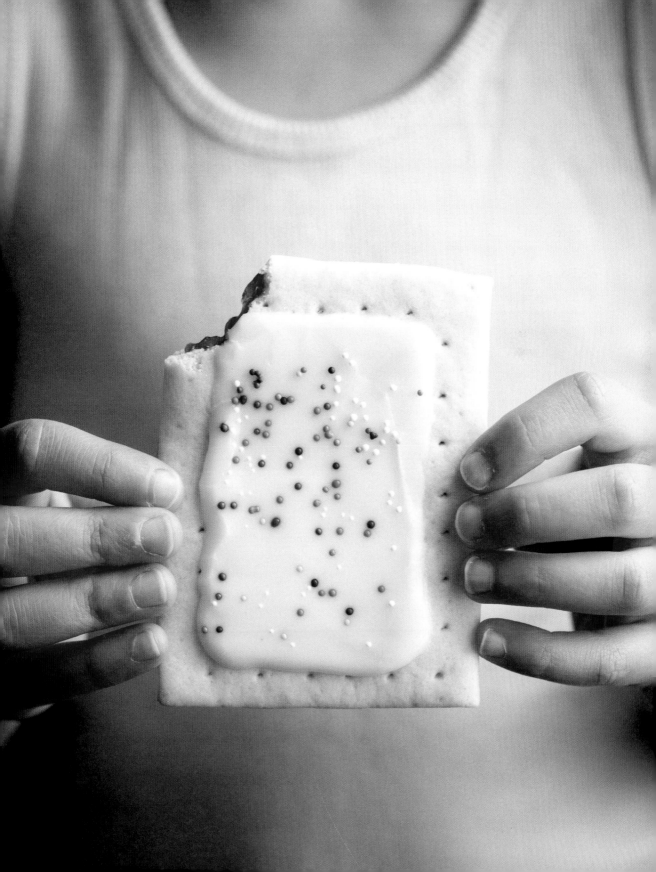

Kellogg's Frosted Brown Sugar Cinnamon Pop-Tarts Toaster Pastries

MAKES 12 PASTRIES

Crust

2¼ cups (315 g) all-purpose gluten-free flour (see page 2), plus more for sprinkling

¼ cup (36 g) cornstarch

¼ teaspoon kosher salt

¾ cup (150 g) granulated sugar

8 tablespoons (112 g) unsalted butter, melted and cooled

1 teaspoon pure vanilla extract

1 egg (50 g weighed out of shell), at room temperature, beaten

4 to 6 tablespoons (2 to 3 fluid ounces) milk, at room temperature

Filling

1 cup (218 g) packed light brown sugar

2 tablespoons (28 g) unsalted butter, melted and cooled

*E*ven with all the many available varieties of Kellogg's Pop-Tarts these days, my heart will forever belong to frosted brown sugar and cinnamon. I think I ate one every morning of my childhood. If you follow my lead and enjoy the Strawberry Frosted variety (page 223) untoasted, then this is the one to toast lightly. The sweet aroma of the brown sugar and cinnamon inside the tender, buttery crust will fill your kitchen. Just be sure to allow the pastry to cool briefly before you touch that frosting—it can get quite hot in the toaster!

Prepare the crust: Preheat your oven to 350°F. Line a large rimmed baking sheet with unbleached parchment paper and set it aside.

In a large bowl, place the flour, cornstarch, salt, and sugar, and whisk to combine well. Create a well in the center of the dry ingredients, and add the butter, vanilla, egg, and 2 fluid ounces of the milk, mixing to combine after each addition. The dough will be thick. Knead the dough with your hands until it is smooth, adding more milk by the half-teaspoonful as necessary to bring the dough together. Place the dough on a lightly floured surface and dust lightly with flour to prevent the dough from sticking to the rolling pin. Roll out the dough ¼ inch thick and slice it into 3½ x 4½-inch rectangles. Gather and reroll any scraps, and cut out as many more rectangles as possible (it should be at least twenty-four rectangles). If the dough becomes difficult to handle at any point, wrap it in plastic wrap and place it in the freezer to chill briefly.

Prepare the filling: In a medium-size bowl, place all the filling ingredients and mix until smooth. Place 1 tablespoon of filling on the center of half of the rectangles of dough, and spread into an even layer, leaving a ¾-inch border clean on all sides of the rectangle. Cover with the remaining rectangles of dough and press all around the clean edge to seal. Using a sharp knife or pastry or pizza wheel, cut off about ½ inch of dough around all sides of each pastry. Place the pastries about 2 inches apart from one another on the prepared baking sheet. Dock the pastries by piercing randomly on top with a toothpick or wooden skewer. Place the baking sheet in the center of the preheated oven and bake until the pastries are very lightly golden brown around the edges and just set in the center, about 8 minutes.

Remove from the oven and allow to cool on the baking sheet for 10 minutes before transferring to a wire rack to cool completely.

While the pastries are cooling, prepare the glaze: In a medium-size bowl, place the confectioners' sugar, brown sugar, and 1 tablespoon of the water, and mix until combined into a thick paste. Add more water by the half-teaspoonful as necessary to create a thickly pourable glaze. Spread the glaze thickly on top of each cooled pastry. Allow to set at room temperature before serving.

The finished pastries can be stored in a sealed glass container at room temperature and should maintain their texture for at least 3 days. For longer storage, wrap individually in freezer-safe wrap, and freeze for up to 2 months. Defrost at room temperature or unwrap and defrost in the toaster.

⅛ teaspoon kosher salt

½ teaspoon ground cinnamon

Glaze

1½ cups (173 g) confectioners' sugar

¼ cup (55 g) packed light brown sugar

1 tablespoon (½ fluid ounce) lukewarm water, plus more by the half-teaspoonful

Kellogg's Frosted Chocolate Fudge Pop-Tarts Toaster Pastries

MAKES 12 PASTRIES

Crust

2¼ cups (315 g) all-purpose gluten-free flour (see page 2), plus more for sprinkling

½ cup + 2 tablespoons (50 g) unsweetened cocoa powder

¼ teaspoon kosher salt

¾ cup (150 g) granulated sugar

8 tablespoons (112 g) unsalted butter, at room temperature

1 tablespoon (14 g) canola oil

1 teaspoon pure vanilla extract

1 egg (50 g, weighed out of shell), at room temperature, beaten

4 to 6 tablespoons (2 to 3 fluid ounces) milk, at room temperature

*Y*ou know how sometimes the manufacturer of a snack food will claim that it has fudge in it, but really it's just chocolate (no fudge)? Well, the light and tender chocolate pastry really *does* give way to a filling with the taste and texture of fudge (the secret ingredient? Cream cheese). The light dusting of coarse sugar on top is, of course, purely optional and mostly for effect. They're plenty sweet without it!

Prepare the crust: Preheat your oven to 350°F. Line a large rimmed baking sheet with unbleached parchment paper and set it aside.

In a large bowl, place the flour, cocoa powder, salt, and sugar, and whisk to combine well. Create a well in the center of the dry ingredients, and add the butter, oil, vanilla, egg, and 2 fluid ounces of the milk, mixing to combine after each addition. The dough will be thick. Knead the dough with your hands until it is smooth, adding more milk by the half-teaspoonful as necessary to bring the dough together. Place the dough on a lightly floured surface and dust lightly with flour to prevent the dough from sticking to the rolling pin. Roll the dough out ¼ inch thick and slice it into 3½ x 4½-inch rectangles. Gather and reroll any scraps, and cut out as many more rectangles as possible (it should be at least twenty-four rectangles). If the dough becomes difficult to handle at any point, wrap it in plastic wrap and place it in the freezer to chill briefly.

Prepare the filling: In a medium-size bowl, place all the filling ingredients and mix until smooth. Place 1 tablespoon of filling on the center of half of the rectangles of dough, and spread into an even layer, leaving a ¾-inch border clean on all sides of the rectangle. Cover with the remaining rectangles of dough and press all around the clean edge to seal. Using a sharp knife or pastry or pizza wheel, cut off about ½ inch of dough around all sides of each pastry. Place the pastries about 2 inches apart from one another on the prepared baking sheets. Dock the pastries by piercing randomly on top with a toothpick or wooden skewer. Place the baking sheet in the center of the preheated oven and bake until the pastries are just set in the center, about 8 minutes.

Remove from the oven and allow to cool on the baking sheet for 10 minutes before transferring to a wire rack to cool completely.

While the pastries are cooling, prepare the glaze: In a medium-size bowl, place the confectioners' sugar, cocoa powder, and 3 tablespoons of the water, and mix until combined into a thick paste. Add more water by the half-teaspoonful as necessary to create a thickly pourable glaze. Spread the glaze thickly on top of each cooled pastry, and sprinkle lightly with coarse sugar, if desired. Allow to set at room temperature before serving.

The finished pastries can be stored in a sealed glass container at room temperature and should maintain their texture for at least 3 days. For longer storage, wrap individually in freezer-safe wrap, and freeze for up to 2 months. Defrost at room temperature or unwrap and defrost in the toaster.

Filling

4 ounces chopped semisweet chocolate, melted and cooled slightly

4 ounces cream cheese

⅓ cup (38 g) confectioners' sugar

Glaze

1½ cups (173 g) confectioners' sugar

4 tablespoons (20 g) unsweetened cocoa powder

3 to 4 tablespoons (1½ to 2 fluid ounces) lukewarm water

Coarse sugar, for sprinkling

Kellogg's Gone Nutty! Frosted Chocolate Peanut Butter Pop-Tarts Toaster Pastries

MAKES 12 PASTRIES

Crust

2¼ cups (315 g) all-purpose gluten-free flour (see page 2), plus more for sprinkling

½ cup + 2 tablespoons (50 g) unsweetened cocoa powder

¼ teaspoon kosher salt

¾ cup (150 g) granulated sugar

8 tablespoons (112 g) unsalted butter, at room temperature

1 tablespoon (14 g) canola oil

1 teaspoon pure vanilla extract

1 egg (50 g, weighed out of shell), at room temperature, beaten

4 to 6 tablespoons (2 to 3 fluid ounces) milk, at room temperature

*J*f you were hoping to convince yourself that Pop-Tarts are, in fact, viable as a "proper breakfast," the frosted chocolate peanut butter pastry is where that illusion probably breaks down entirely. These taste like a cross between chocolate pie and a peanut butter cup. They might be a bit sinful, but if that's wrong, it also might just be what makes them taste even better. As with other recipes in this book that call for peanut butter, a no-stir variety (the kind that doesn't separate) performs best.

Prepare the crust: Preheat your oven to 350°F. Line a large rimmed baking sheet with unbleached parchment paper and set it aside.

In a large bowl, place the flour, cocoa powder, salt, and sugar, and whisk to combine well. Create a well in the center of the dry ingredients, and add the butter, oil, vanilla, egg, and 2 fluid ounces of the milk, mixing to combine after each addition. The dough will be thick. Knead the dough with your hands until it is smooth, adding more milk by the half-teaspoonful as necessary to bring the dough together. Place the dough on a lightly floured surface and dust lightly with flour to prevent the dough from sticking to the rolling pin. Roll out the dough ¼ inch thick and slice it into 3½ x 4½-inch rectangles. Gather and reroll any scraps, and cut out as many more rectangles as possible (it should be at least twenty-four rectangles). If the dough becomes difficult to handle at any point, wrap it in plastic wrap and place it in the freezer to chill briefly.

Prepare the filling: In a medium-size bowl, place both filling ingredients and mix until smooth. Place 1 tablespoon of filling on the center of half of the rectangles of dough, and spread into an even layer, leaving a ¾-inch border clean on all sides of the rectangle. Cover with the remaining rectangles of dough and press all around the clean edge to seal.

Using a sharp knife or pastry or pizza wheel, cut off about ½ inch of dough around all sides of each pastry. Place the pastries about 2 inches apart from one another on the prepared baking sheet. Dock the pastries by piercing randomly on top with a toothpick or wooden skewer. Place the baking sheet in the center of the preheated oven and bake until the pastries are just set in the center, about 8 minutes.

Remove from the oven and allow to cool on the baking sheet for 10 minutes before transferring to a wire rack to cool completely.

While the pastries are cooling, make the glaze: In a medium-size bowl, place the confectioners' sugar, cocoa powder, and 3 tablespoons of the water, and mix until combined into a thick paste. Add more water by the half-teaspoonful as necessary to create a thick, pourable glaze. Spread the glaze thickly on top of each cooled pastry. Allow to set at room temperature before serving.

The finished pastries can be stored in a sealed glass container at room temperature and should maintain their texture for at least 3 days. For longer storage, wrap individually in freezer-safe wrap, and freeze for up to 2 months. Defrost at room temperature or unwrap and defrost in the toaster.

Filling

½ cup (128 g) smooth, no-stir peanut butter, melted

⅓ cup (38 g) confectioners' sugar

Glaze

1½ cups (173 g) confectioners' sugar

4 tablespoons (20 g) unsweetened cocoa powder

3 to 4 tablespoons (1½ to 2 fluid ounces) lukewarm water

Quaker Chewy Granola Bars, Oatmeal Raisin

MAKES 12 BARS

3 cups (300 g) certified gluten-free old-fashioned rolled oats

¾ cup (60 g) coconut flakes

1½ cups (45 g) gluten-free crisp rice cereal

3 tablespoons plus 1 teaspoon (20 g) nonfat dry milk, ground into a finer powder

¼ cup (36 g) all-purpose gluten-free flour (see page 2)

⅛ teaspoon kosher salt

⅛ teaspoon baking soda

1 teaspoon ground cinnamon

5 tablespoons (70 g) unsalted butter, chopped

¼ cup (55 g) packed light brown sugar

½ cup (168 g) Lyle's golden syrup

½ cup (168 g) light corn syrup

5 ounces raisins

A touch of cinnamon and raisins instead of miniature chocolate chips are all it takes to transform these chewy granola bars into a variety with an entirely different taste from the bars on page 234. If you're thinking of replacing the refined sugars here with unrefined ones, check out the headnote for Quaker Chewy Granola Bars, Chocolate Chip for tips!

Preheat your oven to 275°F. Line an 8-inch square pan with two sheets of unbleached parchment paper, crisscrossed in the pan, with enough paper to overhang the edges, and set it aside.

Line a large rimmed baking sheet with unbleached parchment paper, and place the oats and coconut flakes on it. Shake the oats and coconut into an even layer, and place in the preheated oven. Bake until the oats and coconut are just beginning to brown and the oats are becoming fragrant, taking care not to let them burn, about 7 minutes. Remove from the oven and transfer to a large bowl. Add the rice cereal, nonfat dry milk, flour, salt, baking soda, and cinnamon, and mix to combine well. Set the bowl aside.

In a small, heavy-bottomed saucepan, place the butter, brown sugar, golden syrup, and corn syrup, and melt over medium-low heat, stirring occasionally, until smooth. Pour the melted butter and sugar mixture into the bowl of dry ingredients and mix to combine well, making sure to moisten all the dry ingredients with the wet ingredients. Add 4 ounces of the raisins, reserving 1 ounce.

Scrape the mixture into the prepared square baking pan and press down very firmly and evenly to compress the granola bars into a very compact, even layer in the pan. It can be very helpful to place a piece of plastic wrap on top of the granola bars, then place another 8-inch baking pan on top and press down on the empty pan to compress the bars evenly. Remove the top baking pan and the plastic wrap, and scatter the remaining raisins evenly on top. Press the raisins gently into the top of the bars with a spatula. Cover the baking pan with plastic wrap and refrigerate for at least 2 hours, or until very firm. Remove from the refrigerator, lift out of the pan by holding onto the parchment paper, and slice into twelve equal rectangular bars.

These bars are somewhat sticky, but they are very stable. It is best to wrap each of them separately in plastic wrap after they are sliced into bars and store them at room temperature for up to a week. For longer storage, seal tightly in a freezer-safe bag, and freeze for up to 2 months. Defrost at room temperature.

Quaker Chewy Granola Bars, Chocolate Chip

MAKES 12 BARS

3 cups (300 g) certified gluten-free old-fashioned rolled oats

¾ cup (60 g) coconut flakes

1½ cups (45 g) gluten-free crisp rice cereal

3 tablespoons plus 1 teaspoon (20 g) nonfat dry milk, ground into a finer powder

¼ cup (36 g) all-purpose gluten-free flour (see page 2)

⅛ teaspoon kosher salt

⅛ teaspoon baking soda

5 tablespoons (70 g) unsalted butter, chopped

¼ cup (55 g) packed light brown sugar

½ cup (168 g) Lyle's golden syrup

½ cup (168 g) light corn syrup

5 ounces miniature chocolate chips

These perfectly chewy granola bars are not baked, and the honest truth of it all is that they hold together well anyway . . . because of the sugars. I tried making them with less sugar, and they simply fell apart. I tried making them with unrefined sugars and they were delicious, but they simply did not taste like Quaker Chewy Granola Bars. So if you don't mind a nice, chewy granola bar that doesn't taste like the "real thing," go ahead and replace both the Lyle's golden syrup and the corn syrup with an equal amount of honey and the brown sugar with an equal amount of coconut palm sugar. But you might want to make them as written at least once, just to see how much they taste like the real deal: chewy, oaty, sticky, and coconutty, with the light chocolate taste of miniature chocolate chips throughout!

Preheat your oven to 275°F. Line an 8-inch square pan with two sheets of unbleached parchment paper, crisscrossed in the pan, with enough paper to overhang the edges, and set it aside.

Line a large rimmed baking sheet with unbleached parchment paper, and place the oats and coconut flakes on it. Shake the oats and coconut into an even layer, and place in the preheated oven. Bake until the oats and coconut are just beginning to brown and the oats are becoming fragrant, taking care not to let them burn, about 7 minutes. Remove from the oven and transfer to a large bowl. Add the rice cereal, nonfat dry milk, flour, salt, and baking soda, and mix to combine well. Set the bowl aside.

In a small, heavy-bottomed saucepan, place the butter, brown sugar, golden syrup, and corn syrup, and melt over medium-low heat, stirring occasionally, until smooth. Pour the melted butter and sugar mixture into the bowl of dry ingredients and mix to combine well, making sure to moisten all the dry ingredients with the wet ingredients. Allow the mixture to cool until it is no longer hot to the touch, and add 4 ounces of the mini chocolate chips, reserving 1 ounce.

Scrape the mixture into the prepared square baking pan and press down very firmly and evenly to compress the granola bars into a very compact, even layer in the pan. It can be very helpful to place a piece of plastic wrap on top of the granola bars, then place another 8-inch baking pan on top and press down on the empty pan to compress the bars evenly. Remove the top baking pan and the plastic wrap, and scatter the remaining chocolate chips on top. Press the chips gently into the top of the bars with a spatula. Cover the baking pan with plastic wrap and refrigerate for at least 2 hours, or until very firm. Remove from the refrigerator, lift out of the pan by holding onto the parchment paper, and slice into twelve equal rectangular bars.

These bars are somewhat sticky, but they are very stable. It is best to wrap each of them separately in plastic wrap after they are sliced into bars and store them at room temperature for up to a week. For longer storage, seal tightly in a freezer-safe bag, and freeze for up to 2 months. Defrost at room temperature.

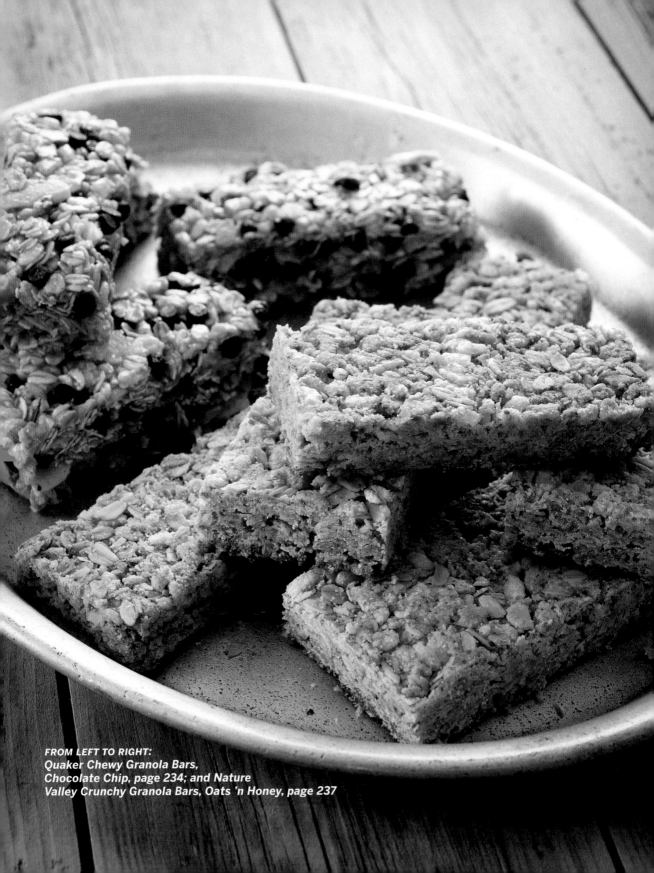

FROM LEFT TO RIGHT:
Quaker Chewy Granola Bars,
Chocolate Chip, page 234; and Nature
Valley Crunchy Granola Bars, Oats 'n Honey, page 237

Nature Valley Crunchy Granola Bars, Oats 'n Honey

MAKES 15 BARS

*T*hese crunchy bars look (see for yourself) and taste (take my word for it for now) just like the original: crispy, crunchy, and nutty, with the full-bodied taste of honey. The almond flour can be replaced with an equal amount, by weight, of cashew flour or sunflower seed flour. You can buy either flour already ground at Nuts.com (see Resources, page 296) or buy whole raw cashews or shelled sunflower seeds from the same source and grind your own.

Preheat your oven to 325°F. Line a quarter sheet (13 x 9 x 1-inch) pan with unbleached parchment paper and set it aside.

In a large bowl, place the almond flour, salt, and sugar, and whisk to combine well. Add the oats and rice cereal, and then the honey and oil, and mix to combine well.

Scrape the mixture onto the prepared baking sheet and spread into an even layer. Cover the baking sheet with another sheet of unbleached parchment paper, and place another quarter sheet pan on top of the top sheet of parchment paper. Apply as much even pressure as possible on the top sheet pan to compress the mixture as much as possible.

Remove the top quarter sheet pan and the top piece of parchment paper, and place the baking sheet in the center of the preheated oven. Bake for about 25 minutes, or until the bars are evenly golden brown.

Remove the baking sheet from the oven and allow the bars cool for 5 minutes before lifting up on the parchment paper and placing the bars on a cutting board. Slice into three rows of five rectangles. Allow to cool completely before separating the bars. They will crisp as they cool and will hold together well once cool.

These can be stored in a sealed glass or plastic container at room temperature and should maintain their texture for about 5 days. For longer storage, wrap individually in freezer-safe wrap, and freeze for up to 2 months. Defrost at room temperature.

---

1 cup (120 g) almond flour

½ teaspoon kosher salt

½ cup (100 g) granulated sugar

2 cups (200 g) certified gluten-free old-fashioned rolled oats

2 cups (60 g) gluten-free crisp rice cereal

6 tablespoons (126 g) honey

5 tablespoons (70 g) virgin coconut oil, melted

Nature Valley Crunchy Granola Bars, Apple Crisp

MAKES 15 BARS

¾ cup (90 g) almond flour

2 cups (55 g) freeze-dried apples, ground into a powder

½ teaspoon kosher salt

1 teaspoon ground cinnamon

½ cup (100 g) granulated sugar

1¾ cups (175 g) certified gluten-free old-fashioned rolled oats

2 cups (60 g) gluten-free crisp rice cereal

6 tablespoons (126 g) honey

5 tablespoons (70 g) virgin coconut oil, melted

Freeze-dried fruit is so useful in baking, as it adds flavor without upsetting the moisture balance in the recipe at all. Just Tomatoes, Etc.! brand of freeze-dried fruits and vegetables is available in large grocery stores. I grind them into a powder in a blender or food processor. If you're looking to replace the almond flour in this recipe, see the headnote for the Oats 'n Honey variety (page 237).

Preheat your oven to 325°F. Line a quarter sheet (13 x 9 x 1-inch) pan with unbleached parchment paper and set it aside.

In a large bowl, place the almond flour, ground dried apples, salt, cinnamon, and sugar, and whisk to combine well. Add the oats and rice cereal, and then the honey and oil, and mix to combine well.

Scrape the mixture onto the prepared baking sheet and spread into an even layer. Cover the baking sheet with another sheet of unbleached parchment paper, and place another quarter sheet pan on top of the top sheet of parchment paper. Apply as much even pressure as possible on the top sheet pan to compress the mixture as much as possible.

Remove the top quarter sheet pan and the top piece of parchment paper, and place the baking sheet in the center of the preheated oven. Bake for about 25 minutes, or until the bars are evenly golden brown.

Remove the baking sheet from the oven and allow the bars cool for 5 minutes before lifting up on the parchment paper and placing the bars on a cutting board. Slice into three rows of five rectangles. Allow to cool completely before separating the bars. They will crisp as they cool and will hold together well once cool.

These can be stored in a sealed glass or plastic container at room temperature and should maintain their texture for about 5 days. For longer storage, wrap individually in freezer-safe wrap, and freeze for up to 2 months. Defrost at room temperature.

Vitalicious VitaMuffin VitaTops, Chocolate Chip

MAKES 12 MUFFIN TOPS

Like Fiber One bars (pages 249–251), VitaTops muffin tops are made with inulin as a way to increase fiber and reduce calories from sugar. I use Swerve sweetener (see page 16 for a description and possible substitutions), a blend of erythritol and inulin. Swerve is nonglycemic and noncaloric but not a significant source of fiber as is the inulin in VitaTops. Although these moist and tender, sweet little chocolate chip–studded cakes don't boast the same vitamin enrichment as the original, they also don't have any of the preservatives. I don't own a muffin top pan (no more pans!), so I make these in my USA Pans six-well cake panel pan, which makes the perfectly sized muffin top. And this is the good kind of muffin top. Not the kind you get when your jeans are too tight.

Preheat your oven to 350°F. Grease the wells of a miniature cake panel pan or muffin top pan, and set it aside. A standard twelve-cup muffin tin can also be used instead to make regular-size muffins.

In a large bowl, place the all-purpose flour, oat flour, nonfat dry milk, baking soda, baking powder, salt, and Swerve, and whisk to combine well. Transfer 1 teaspoon of the dry ingredients to a small bowl and toss them with the chocolate chips. Set the chips aside. Create a well in the center of the dry ingredients and add the egg whites, coconut oil, molasses, and water, mixing to combine after each addition. Add 3 ounces of the dry ingredients–dusted chocolate chips to the batter, and mix until the chips are evenly distributed throughout. Fill the wells of the prepared pan about one-third full, and shake into an even layer in each well.

Place the pan in the center of the preheated oven and bake for 8 minutes (bake for 5 minutes if using a standard twelve-cup muffin tin).

---

1 cup (140 g) all-purpose gluten-free flour (see page 2)

½ cup (60 g) certified gluten-free oat flour

7 tablespoons (42 g) nonfat dry milk, ground into a finer powder

½ teaspoon baking soda

1 teaspoon baking powder

½ teaspoon kosher salt

¾ cup (180 g) granulated Swerve

4 ounces semisweet chocolate chips

3 egg whites (75 g), at room temperature

4 tablespoons (56 g) virgin coconut oil, melted and cooled

2 tablespoons (42 g) unsulfured molasses

1 cup (8 fluid ounces) warm water

Remove from the oven quickly, sprinkle the remaining ounce of chips evenly over the tops, and return to the oven. Bake until a toothpick inserted into the center of a muffin top comes out clean, 2 to 4 minutes more. Remove from the oven and allow to cool in the pan for 10 minutes, or until firm. Transfer to a wire rack to cool completely. Repeat with the remaining batter.

These can be stored in a sealed glass or plastic container at room temperature and should maintain their texture for about 5 days. For longer storage, wrap individually in freezer-safe wrap, and freeze for up to 2 months. Defrost at room temperature.

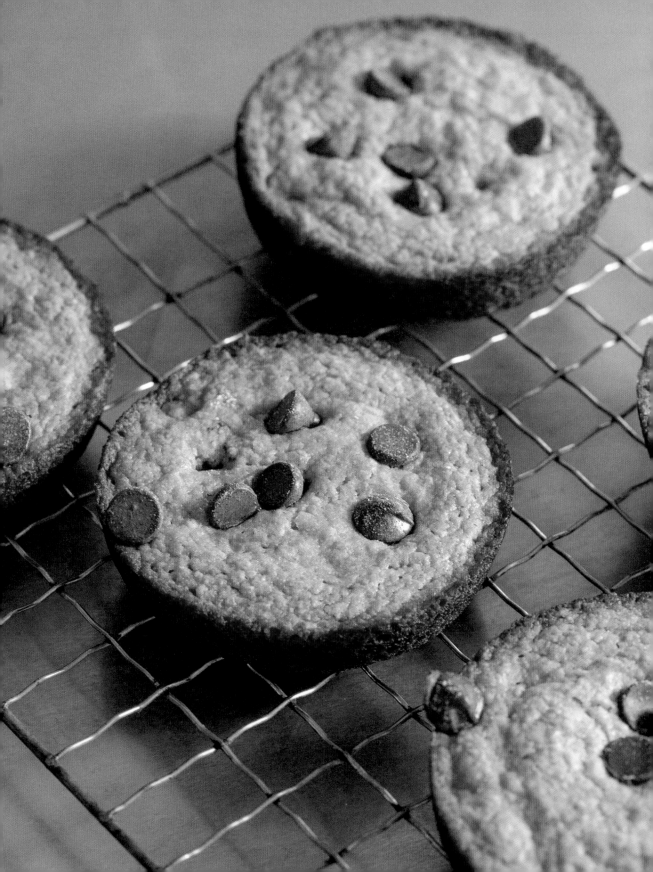

Vitalicious VitaMuffin VitaTops, Blueberry

MAKES 12 MUFFIN TOPS

1 cup (140 g) all-purpose gluten-free flour (see page 2)

½ cup (60 g) certified gluten-free oat flour

7 tablespoons (42 g) nonfat dry milk, ground into a finer powder

½ teaspoon baking soda

1 teaspoon baking powder

½ teaspoon kosher salt

¾ cup (180 g) granulated Swerve

1 cup (80 g) fresh blueberries

3 egg whites (75 g), at room temperature

¼ cup (56 g) virgin coconut oil, melted and cooled

2 tablespoons (42 g) honey

1 cup (8 fluid ounces) warm water

*A*s with the other VitaTops recipes in this chapter, these blueberry muffin tops are more "Top" than "Vita," as they don't have extra vitamins added like the original, but they're also preservative-free. As with most blueberry baking recipes, you can replace the fresh blueberries in this recipe with frozen berries. If using frozen berries, toss them, still frozen, in the dry ingredients as directed for fresh berries in the recipe. Unlike when baking with fresh blueberries, the color of frozen blueberries will always run when you fold them into the batter. It doesn't affect the taste one bit, though! With a touch of honey instead of molasses in the batter, these have a slightly lighter taste than the chocolate chip VitaTops (page 239). For a discussion of the no-calorie, nonglycemic Swerve sweetener in this and the other VitaTops-style recipes, plus possible substitutions, see page 16.

Preheat your oven to 350°F. Grease the wells of a miniature cake panel pan or muffin top pan, and set it aside. A standard twelve-cup muffin tin can also be used instead to make regular-size muffins.

In a large bowl, place the all-purpose flour, oat flour, nonfat dry milk, baking soda, baking powder, salt, and Swerve, and whisk to combine well. Transfer 1 teaspoon of the dry ingredients to a small bowl and toss them with the blueberries. Set the berries aside. Create a well in the center of the dry ingredients and add the egg whites, coconut oil, honey, and water, mixing to combine after each addition. Add ¾ cup (60 g) of the dry ingredients–dusted blueberries to the batter, and fold in gently until the berries are evenly distributed throughout. Fill the wells of the prepared pan about one-third full, and shake into an even layer in each well.

Place the pan in the center of the preheated oven and bake for 8 minutes (bake for 5 minutes if using a standard twelve-cup muffin tin). Remove from the oven quickly, sprinkle the remaining ¼ cup of the blueberries evenly over the tops, and return to the oven. Bake until a toothpick inserted into the center of a muffin top comes out clean, 2 to 4 minutes more. Remove from the oven and allow to cool in the pan for 10 minutes, or until firm. Transfer to a wire rack to cool completely. Repeat with the remaining batter.

These can be stored in a sealed glass or plastic container at room temperature and should maintain their texture for about 5 days. For longer storage, wrap individually in freezer-safe wrap, and freeze for up to 2 months. Defrost at room temperature.

Vitalicious VitaMuffin VitaTops, Deep Chocolate

MAKES 12 MUFFIN TOPS

¾ cup (105 g) all-purpose gluten-free flour (see page 2)

7 tablespoons (35 g) unsweetened cocoa powder

½ cup (60 g) certified gluten-free oat flour

7 tablespoons (42 g) nonfat dry milk, ground into a finer powder

½ teaspoon baking soda

1 teaspoon baking powder

½ teaspoon kosher salt

¾ cup (180 g) granulated Swerve

4 ounces semisweet chocolate chips

3 egg whites (75 g), at room temperature

¼ cup (56 g) virgin coconut oil, melted and cooled

2 tablespoons (42 g) unsulfured molasses

1 cup (8 fluid ounces) warm water

*D*eeply rich and chocolaty, even without any melted chocolate in the batter, these deep chocolate muffin tops are my personal favorite variety. Serve them to your kids, and they'll think they just had chocolate cake for breakfast—but you'll know better. Like the other VitaTops-style muffin top recipes, they're not overly sweet at all (for a full description and potential substitutes for Swerve sweetener, please see page 16), and they don't have the same artificial vitamin enrichment, but they're super satisfying and they'll keep you going all morning long!

Preheat your oven to 350°F. Grease the wells of a miniature cake panel pan or muffin top pan, and set it aside. A standard twelve-cup muffin tin can also be used instead to make regular-size muffins.

In a large bowl, place the all-purpose flour, cocoa powder, oat flour, nonfat dry milk, baking soda, baking powder, salt, and Swerve, and whisk to combine well. Transfer 1 teaspoon of the dry ingredients to a small bowl and toss them with the chocolate chips. Set the chips aside. Create a well in the center of the dry ingredients and add the egg whites, coconut oil, molasses, and water, mixing to combine after each addition. Add 3 ounces of the dry ingredients—dusted chocolate chips to the batter, and mix until the chips are evenly distributed throughout. Fill the wells of the prepared pan about one-third full, and shake into an even layer in each well.

Place the pan in the center of the preheated oven and bake for 8 minutes (bake for 5 minutes if using a standard twelve-cup muffin tin). Remove from the oven quickly, sprinkle the remaining ounce of chips evenly over the tops, and return to the oven. Bake until a toothpick inserted into the center of a muffin top comes out clean, 2 to 4 minutes more. Remove from the oven and allow to cool in the pan for 10 minutes, or until firm. Transfer to a wire rack to cool completely. Repeat with the remaining batter.

These can be stored in a sealed glass or plastic container at room temperature and should maintain their texture for about 5 days. For longer storage, wrap individually in freezer-safe wrap, and freeze for up to 2 months. Defrost at room temperature.

Vitalicious VitaMuffin VitaTops, Banana Chocolate Chip

MAKES 12 MUFFIN TOPS

1 cup (140 g) all-purpose gluten-free flour (see page 2)

½ cup (60 g) certified gluten-free oat flour

7 tablespoons (42 g) nonfat dry milk, ground into a finer powder

½ teaspoon baking soda

1 teaspoon baking powder

½ teaspoon kosher salt

½ cup (120 g) granulated Swerve

4 ounces semisweet chocolate chips

¾ cup (75 g) certified gluten-free old-fashioned rolled oats

3 egg whites (75 g), at room temperature

2 tablespoons (28 g) virgin coconut oil, melted and cooled

1 medium-size ripe banana (100 g), mashed

The mashed ripe banana in this recipe adds tons of flavor and moisture and allows us to cut back on the coconut oil by half. If you love tender, sweet banana cake, you'll love these muffin tops. See page 16 for a discussion about the Swerve sugar-free sweetener in this recipe. Remember, like the other VitaTops-style recipes, they're not artificially enriched with extra vitamins, but they're also preservative-free.

Preheat your oven to 350°F. Grease the wells of a miniature cake panel pan or muffin top pan, and set it aside. A standard twelve-cup muffin tin can also be used instead to make regular-size muffins.

In a large bowl, place the all-purpose flour, oat flour, nonfat dry milk, baking soda, baking powder, salt, and Swerve, and whisk to combine well. Transfer 1 teaspoon of the dry ingredients to a small bowl and toss them with the chocolate chips. Set the chips aside. Add the oats to the bowl of dry ingredients, and mix to combine well. Create a well in the center of the dry ingredients and add the egg whites, coconut oil, mashed banana, molasses, and water, mixing to combine after each addition. Add 3 ounces of the dry ingredients–dusted chocolate chips to the batter, and mix until the chips are evenly distributed throughout. Fill the wells of the prepared pan about one-third full, and shake into an even layer in each well.

Place the pan in the center of the preheated oven and bake for 8 minutes (bake for 5 minutes if using a standard twelve-cup muffin tin). Remove from the oven quickly, sprinkle the remaining ounce of chips evenly over the tops, and return to the oven. Bake until a toothpick inserted into the center of a muffin top comes out clean, 2 to 4 minutes more. Remove from the oven and allow to cool in the pan for 10 minutes, or until firm. Transfer to a wire rack to cool completely. Repeat with the remaining batter.

These can be stored in a sealed glass or plastic container at room temperature and should maintain their texture for about 5 days. For longer storage, wrap individually in freezer-safe wrap, and freeze for up to 2 months. Defrost at room temperature.

1 tablespoon (21 g) unsulfured molasses

¾ cup (6 fluid ounces) warm water

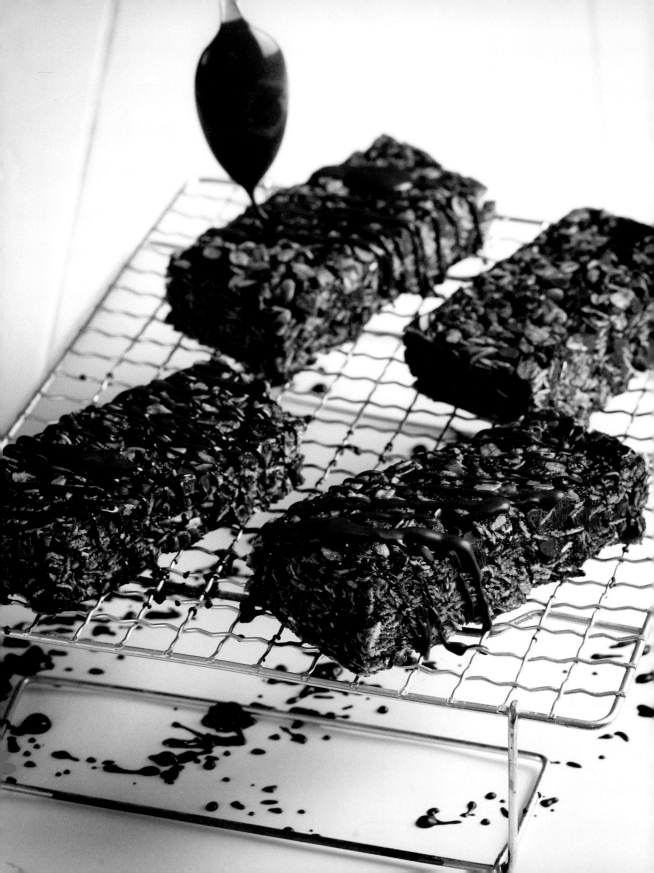

Fiber One Chewy Bars, Oats and Chocolate

MAKES 12 BARS

$\mathcal{G}$et your pencils ready and your glasses on. Chemistry class is in session! Nah, just kidding. We'll keep this pretty basic, but I want you to understand the what and the why of the recipe ingredients in these Fiber One bars. The first ingredient in "real" Fiber One bars is chicory root extract, which is a significant source of fiber. This recipe calls for Swerve brand sweetener (see page 16), which is a blend of erythritol (a sugar alcohol) and oligosaccharides, of which inulin (chicory root) is one. The best thing about Swerve is that it's nonglycemic and noncaloric. Keep in mind, though, that according to Swerve, its sweeteners are not a significant source of fiber, so these bars don't boast the same fiber content as the actual Fiber One bars. But they do have fewer calories gram for gram than the original (these homemade bars are more than twice the size of the packaged original). The bottom line? These bars are very satisfying and plenty sweet with just a touch of actual sugar. Class dismissed!

Preheat your oven to 350°F. Grease and line an 8-inch square pan with two sheets of unbleached parchment paper, crisscrossed in the pan, with enough paper to overhang the edges, and set it aside.

In a large bowl, place the flour, cocoa powder, salt, baking soda, nonfat dry milk, and Swerve, and whisk to combine well. Add the oats and mix to combine. Create a well in the center of the dry ingredients and add the molasses, corn syrup, shortening, and oil, mixing to combine well after each addition. Add the chocolate chips, and mix until the chips are evenly distributed throughout. Scrape the mixture into the prepared baking pan, and press firmly into an even layer.

Place the pan in the center of the preheated oven and bake until the bars are mostly firm to the touch, about 12 minutes. Remove from the

¼ cup (35 g) all-purpose gluten-free flour (see page 2)

3 tablespoons (15 g) unsweetened cocoa powder

¼ teaspoon kosher salt

⅛ teaspoon baking soda

3 tablespoons plus 1 teaspoon (20 g) nonfat dry milk, ground into a finer powder

1 cup (240 g) granulated Swerve

3 cups (300 g) certified gluten-free old-fashioned rolled oats

2 tablespoons (42 g) unsulfured molasses

4 tablespoons (84 g) light corn syrup

4 tablespoons (48 g) nonhydrogenated vegetable shortening, melted and cooled

4 tablespoons (56 g) canola oil

CONTINUED ON PAGE 250

CONTINUED FROM PAGE 249

4 ounces miniature chocolate chips

3 ounces semisweet chocolate, chopped, for drizzling

———————

oven and allow to cool in the baking pan for 30 minutes before transferring to a wire rack to cool completely by holding on to the parchment paper and lifting from the pan. Once the bars have cooled, transfer to a cutting board and cut into twelve rectangles with a sharp knife. Return the bars to the wire rack, and place a sheet of parchment or waxed paper beneath the rack.

Melt the chocolate in a small, heat-safe bowl according to the instructions on page 21. Drizzle the melted chocolate on top of the cooled bars, and allow to set at room temperature.

These keep best wrapped separately in plastic wrap after they are sliced into bars and stored at room temperature for up to a week. For longer storage, seal tightly in a freezer-safe bag, and freeze for up to 2 months. Defrost at room temperature.

Fiber One Chewy Bars, Oats and Peanut Butter

MAKES 12 BARS

This peanut butter variety of Fiber One bars is a really satisfying snack for breakfast or for any time of day. My kids love having them for breakfast, and one generous bar will keep them full for hours. And my kids are eaters! To learn about the what and the why of the ingredients in these bars (as well as the relatively lower fiber content of these homemade bars versus the original), chemistry class is always in session in the headnote on page 249. Be sure to use a no-stir peanut butter (the kind that doesn't separate in the jar), such as Skippy Natural Creamy, for drizzling on top.

Preheat your oven to 350°F. Grease and line an 8-inch square pan with two sheets of unbleached parchment paper, crisscrossed in the pan, with enough paper to overhang the edges, and set it aside.

In a large bowl, place the flour, salt, baking soda, nonfat dry milk, and Swerve, and whisk to combine well. Add the oats and mix to combine. Create a well in the center of the dry ingredients and add the corn syrup, shortening, and oil, mixing to combine well after each addition. Add the peanut butter chips and roasted peanuts, and mix until they are evenly distributed throughout. Scrape the mixture into the prepared baking pan, and press firmly into an even layer.

Place the pan in the center of the preheated oven and bake until the bars are mostly firm to the touch, about 12 minutes. Remove from the oven and allow to cool in the baking pan for 30 minutes before transferring to a wire rack to cool completely by holding on to the parchment paper and lifting from the pan. Once the bars have cooled, transfer to a cutting board and cut into twelve rectangles with a sharp knife. Return the bars to the wire rack, and place a sheet of parchment or waxed paper beneath the rack.

Place the peanut butter in a small, heat-safe bowl and melt in the microwave in 30-second bursts, or in a small, heavy-bottomed saucepan

---

⅓ cup (47 g) all-purpose gluten-free flour (see page 2)

¼ teaspoon kosher salt

⅛ teaspoon baking soda

3 tablespoons plus 1 teaspoon (20 g) nonfat dry milk, ground into a finer powder

1 cup (240 g) granulated Swerve

3 cups (300 g) certified gluten-free old-fashioned rolled oats

6 tablespoons (126 g) light corn syrup

4 tablespoons (48 g) nonhydrogenated vegetable shortening, melted and cooled

4 tablespoons (56 g) canola oil

3 ounces peanut butter chips

3 ounces roasted peanuts, chopped

Smooth no-stir peanut butter, for drizzling

---

over medium heat. Drizzle the melted peanut butter on top of the cooled bars, and allow to set at room temperature.

These keep best wrapped separately in plastic wrap after they are sliced into bars and stored at room temperature for up to a week. The peanut butter drizzle on top may smudge. For longer storage, seal tightly in a freezer-safe bag, and freeze for up to 2 months. Defrost at room temperature.

Nabisco Original Fig Newtons

MAKES 24 COOKIES

*F*ig Newtons are the standard-bearer for the whole Newton line of cookies, but the name is no longer "Fig Newtons," apparently. They just go by the name "Newtons," now. I guess it's like when you're growing up and everyone calls you Richie even though your given name is Richard, but at some point you insist upon being called Richard, as it is your name, after all. Regardless, the flavor of your basic Newton is still fig. All that means is that there is a nice, sweet fig paste inside the tender, buttery cookie pastry.

Preheat your oven to 350°F. Line rimmed baking sheets with unbleached parchment paper and set them aside.

In a food processor fitted with a steel blade, place the dried figs and honey. Purée until smooth. The mixture should be thick but spreadable. If it seems too thick to spread, add the water by the tablespoonful and pulse to combine until you reach the desired consistency.

In a large bowl, place the flour, salt, granulated sugar, and brown sugar, and whisk to combine well, working out any lumps. Create a well in the center of the dry ingredients and add the butter, eggs, and vanilla, and mix until the dough comes together. Knead briefly until smooth. Divide the dough in thirds.

Place one third of the dough between two sheets of unbleached parchment paper and roll into a rectangle about 7 x 11 inches, and slightly less than ¼ inch thick. Remove the top sheet of parchment paper and trim any rough edges of the dough with a sharp knife or pizza or pastry wheel, and discard any trimmings.

Place one third of the dried fruit mixture in the center of the first rectangle of dough and spread lengthwise across the center third of the rectangle. Gently lift one long portion of the bottom sheet of parchment paper and use it to fold the dough over the filling. Peel back the parchment paper and repeat with the other side of the dough, overlapping it

2 cups (280 g) dried figs

1 tablespoon (21 g) honey or Lyle's golden syrup

1 to 2 tablespoons (½ to 1 fluid ounce) lukewarm water

2½ cups (350 g) all-purpose gluten-free flour (see page 2)

¼ teaspoon kosher salt

½ cup (100 g) granulated sugar

¼ cup (55 g) packed light brown sugar

8 tablespoons (112 g) unsalted butter, at room temperature

2 eggs (100 g, weighed out of shell), at room temperature, beaten

1 teaspoon pure vanilla extract

on itself. Place the filled dough in the freezer for about 10 minutes, or until firm enough to slice easily. Repeat with the remaining two pieces of dough and remaining two thirds of the filling.

Remove the filled pieces of dough from the freezer and slice each in cross-section into eight cookies of equal size. Place the cookies, seam-side down, about 1 inch apart on the prepared baking sheets. Place the baking sheets in the center of the preheated oven and bake until the cookies are puffed, light golden brown around the edges, and pale golden on top, about 17 minutes. Remove from the oven and allow to cool on the baking sheets for 10 minutes, or until stable, before transferring to a wire rack to cool completely.

These can be stored in a sealed glass or plastic container at room temperature and should maintain their texture for about 5 days. For longer storage, wrap individually in freezer-safe wrap, and freeze for up to 2 months. Defrost at room temperature.

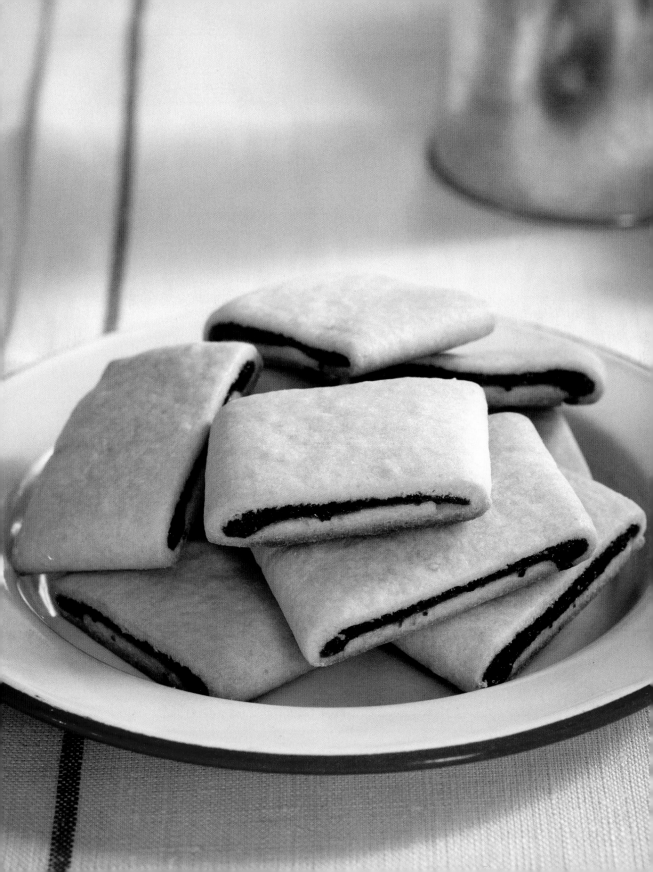

Nabisco Strawberry Newtons

MAKES 24 COOKIES

1½ cups (200 g) dried strawberries

½ cup (80 g) dried prunes

1 tablespoon (21 g) honey or Lyle's golden syrup

1 to 2 tablespoons (½ to 1 fluid ounce) lukewarm water

2½ cups (350 g) all-purpose gluten-free flour (see page 2)

¼ teaspoon kosher salt

½ cup (100 g) granulated sugar

¼ cup (55 g) packed light brown sugar

8 tablespoons (112 g) unsalted butter, at room temperature

2 eggs (100 g, weighed out of shell), at room temperature, beaten

1 teaspoon pure vanilla extract

*T*hese Newtons have a strawberry filling that is actually a blend of prunes and dried strawberries. I find dried strawberries at Nuts.com, and although this is the only reason I order them, they're well worth the special order. If you don't like to special-order dried strawberries and can't find them in your local grocery store, feel free to substitute any other dried fruit in equal measure, by weight, for the strawberries. I buy most of my dried fruits from Nuts.com (see Resources, page 296).

Preheat your oven to 350°F. Line rimmed baking sheets with unbleached parchment paper and set them aside.

In a food processor fitted with a steel blade, place the strawberries, prunes, and honey. Purée until smooth. The mixture should be thick but spreadable. If it seems too thick to spread, add the water by the tablespoon and pulse to combine until you reach the desired consistency.

In a large bowl, place the flour, salt, granulated sugar, and brown sugar, and whisk to combine well, working out any lumps. Create a well in the center of the dry ingredients and add the butter, eggs, and vanilla, and mix until the dough comes together. Knead briefly until smooth. Divide the dough in thirds.

Place one third of the dough between two sheets of unbleached parchment paper and roll into a rectangle about 7 x 11 inches, and slightly less than ¼ inch thick. Remove the top sheet of parchment paper and trim any rough edges of the dough with a sharp knife or pizza or pastry wheel, and discard any trimmings.

Place one third of the dried fruit mixture in the center of the first rectangle of dough and spread lengthwise across the center third of the rectangle. Gently lift one long portion of the bottom sheet of parchment paper and use it to fold the dough over the filling. Peel back the parchment paper and repeat with the other side of the dough, overlapping it on itself. Place the filled dough in the freezer for about 10 minutes, or until firm enough to slice easily. Repeat with the remaining two pieces of dough and remaining two thirds of the filling.

Remove the filled pieces of dough from the freezer and slice each in cross-section into eight cookies of equal size. Place the cookies, seam-side down, about 1 inch apart on the prepared baking sheets. Place the baking sheets in the center of the preheated oven and bake until the cookies are puffed, light golden brown around the edges, and pale golden on top, about 17 minutes. Remove from the oven and allow to cool on the baking sheets for 10 minutes, or until stable, before transferring to a wire rack to cool completely.

These can be stored in a sealed glass or plastic container at room temperature and should maintain their texture for about 5 days. For longer storage, wrap individually in freezer-safe wrap, and freeze for up to 2 months. Defrost at room temperature.

Nabisco 100% Whole Grain Fig Newtons

MAKES 24 COOKIES

2 cups (280 g) dried figs

1 tablespoon (21 g) honey or Lyle's golden syrup

1 to 2 tablespoons (½ to 1 fluid ounce) lukewarm water

1¾ cups (245 g) all-purpose gluten-free flour (see page 2)

¾ cup (105 g) whole-grain gluten-free flour blend (see page 8)

2 tablespoons (18 g) cornstarch

¼ teaspoon kosher salt

½ cup (100 g) granulated sugar

¼ cup (55 g) packed light brown sugar

8 tablespoons (112 g) unsalted butter, at room temperature

2 eggs (100 g, weighed out of shell), at room temperature, beaten

1 teaspoon pure vanilla extract

Lukewarm water by the half-teaspoonful, as necessary

Along with becoming simply "Newtons," the Nabisco people have seen fit to add a few whole-grain varieties to the line. I'm quite glad they did, as the cookie pastry wrapped around the fig paste in this variety has a heartier, satisfying bite that even makes them a bit more healthful. But they're still cookies, so I recommend eating them as such—without counting calories.

Preheat your oven to 350°F. Line rimmed baking sheets with unbleached parchment paper and set them aside.

In a food processor fitted with a steel blade, place the figs and the honey. Purée until smooth. The mixture should be thick but spreadable. If it seems too thick to spread, add the water by the tablespoonful and pulse to combine until you reach the desired consistency.

In a large bowl, place the all-purpose flour, whole-grain flour blend, cornstarch, salt, granulated sugar, and brown sugar, and whisk to combine well, working out any lumps. Create a well in the center of the dry ingredients and add the butter, eggs, and vanilla, and mix until the dough comes together. Knead briefly until smooth, adding water by the half-teaspoonful as necessary to bring the dough together. Divide the dough in thirds.

Place one third of the dough between two sheets of unbleached parchment paper and roll into a rectangle about 7 x 11 inches, and slightly less than ¼ inch thick. Remove the top sheet of parchment paper and trim any rough edges from the dough with a sharp knife or pizza or pastry wheel, and discard any trimmings.

Place one third of the dried fruit mixture in the center of the first rectangle of dough and spread lengthwise across the center third of the rectangle. Gently lift one long portion of the bottom sheet of parchment paper and use it to fold the dough over the filling. Peel back the parchment paper and repeat with the other side of the dough, overlapping it on itself. Place the filled dough in the freezer for about 10 minutes, or until firm enough to slice easily. Repeat with the remaining two pieces of dough and remaining two thirds of the filling.

Remove the filled pieces of dough from the freezer and slice each in cross-section into eight cookies of equal size. Place the cookies, seam-side down about 1 inch apart, on the prepared baking sheets. Place the baking sheets, one at a time, in the center of the preheated oven and bake until the cookies are puffed, light golden brown around the edges, and pale golden on top, about 17 minutes. Remove from the oven and allow to cool on the baking sheets for 10 minutes, or until stable, before transferring to a wire rack to cool completely.

These can be stored in a sealed glass or plastic container at room temperature and should maintain their texture for about 5 days. For longer storage, wrap individually in freezer-safe wrap, and freeze for up to 2 months. Defrost at room temperature.

Entenmann's Devil's Food Donuts

MAKES 18 MINIATURE DONUTS

Donuts

1¾ cups (245 g) all-purpose gluten-free flour (see page 2)

½ cup (40 g) unsweetened cocoa powder

1½ teaspoons baking powder

¼ teaspoon baking soda

½ teaspoon kosher salt

¾ cup (150 g) granulated sugar

2 tablespoons (28 g) unsalted butter, at room temperature

2 tablespoons (28 g) canola oil

1 egg (50 g, weighed out of shell) plus 1 egg white (25 g), at room temperature, beaten

¾ cup (6 fluid ounces) buttermilk, at room temperature

1 teaspoon pure vanilla extract

*Y*ou know how the chocolate on top of this chocolate cake donut always pools a little bit in the middle, over the donut hole? To this day, that's the part that I can't wait to get to when I bite into one of these little beauties. Promise you won't skimp on the glaze when you make these in your own kitchen. The donuts really aren't the same without that chocolate pool.

NOTE: You'll need a mini donut pan or an electric donut maker for this recipe. I much prefer the electric donut maker method (I have the Babycakes mini donut maker, see Resources, page 296) as it bakes the donuts on both sides, which results in perfectly rounded donuts.

First, prepare the donuts: To bake them in an oven, preheat your oven to 350°F. Grease a miniature donut pan, and set it aside. To make them in an electric donut maker, warm the appliance according to the manufacturer's directions.

In a large bowl, place the flour, cocoa powder, baking powder, baking soda, salt, and sugar, and whisk to combine well. Create a well in the center of the dry ingredients and add the butter, oil, egg, egg white, buttermilk, and vanilla, mixing well to combine after each addition. The batter will be thick.

If making the donuts in an oven, fill the prepared donut wells about three-quarters full. Place in the center of the oven and bake for about 10 minutes, or until the donuts are set and a toothpick inserted into the center of a donut comes out clean. Remove from the oven and allow to cool briefly in the pan before transferring to a wire rack to cool completely. Repeat with the remaining batter, if any.

If making the donuts in an electric donut maker, fill the bottom of the donut maker wells completely with batter, then close and secure the lid. Allow to bake for 3 minutes. Open the donut maker and remove the donuts with the remover tool included in the package, the tines of a fork, or a chocolate-dipping tool. Transfer to a wire rack to cool completely. Repeat with the remaining batter.

Once the donuts are completely cool, prepare the glaze: In a small, heat-safe bowl, melt the chocolate and coconut oil according to the instructions on page 21. Allow the chocolate to sit at room temperature until it begins to thicken a bit. Immerse the cooled donuts, one at a time, in the glaze: Press down on the donut with a dipping utensil or fork, then flip it gently in the chocolate. Pull the donut out of the chocolate by slipping the utensil under it and bobbing the donut on the surface of the chocolate a few times before pulling it along the edge of the bowl and carefully placing it on a clean sheet of waxed or parchment paper. Allow the chocolate glaze to set at room temperature.

The finished donuts can be stored in a sealed glass or plastic container at room temperature and should maintain their texture for at least 2 days, although the chocolate frosting may soften. For longer storage, seal the glazed donuts tightly in a freezer-safe wrap or bag, and freeze for up to 2 months. Defrost at room temperature. The chocolate frosting may bloom a bit over time, but it won't affect the taste at all.

Chocolate Glaze

16 ounces semisweet chocolate, chopped

4 tablespoons (56 g) virgin coconut oil

———

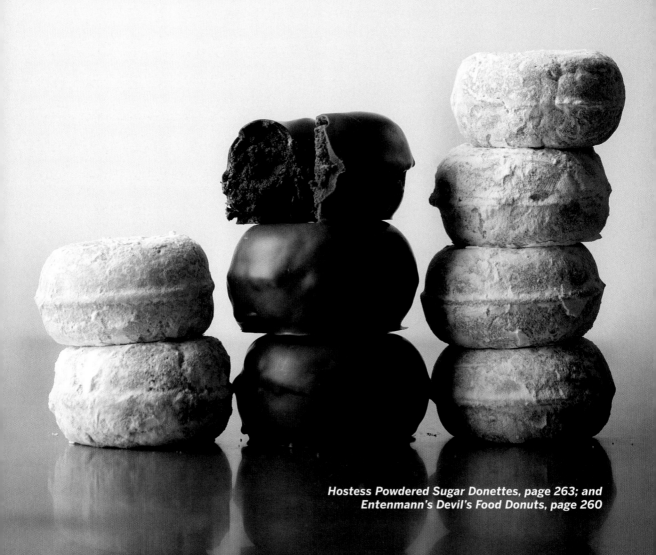

*Hostess Powdered Sugar Donettes, page 263; and
Entenmann's Devil's Food Donuts, page 260*

Hostess Powdered Sugar Donettes

MAKES 18 MINIATURE DONUTS

*P*owdered mini donuts make a mess when you eat them. No matter how gently you try to pick one up with the thumb and forefinger of just one hand, they will immediately shed powdered sugar. That is part of the experience. Don't be like me and try to get your kids to eat them without getting powdered sugar on their nose, fingers, and the floor. You're only setting yourself (and them) up for heartache. Feel free to take big bites and just vacuum afterward!

NOTE: You'll need a mini donut pan or an electric donut maker for this recipe. As discussed in the Entenmann's Devil's Food Donuts (page 260), I prefer the electric donut maker.

To bake the donuts in an oven, preheat your oven to 350°F. Grease a miniature donut pan, and set it aside. To make them in an electric donut maker, warm the appliance according to the manufacturer's directions.

In a large bowl, place the cake flour, baking powder, baking soda, salt, and sugar, and whisk to combine well. Create a well in the center of the dry ingredients and add the butter, egg, egg white, buttermilk, and vanilla, mixing well to combine after each addition. The batter will be thick.

If making the donuts in an oven, fill the prepared donut wells about three-quarters full. Place in the center of the oven and bake for about 10 minutes, or until the donuts are set and a toothpick inserted into the center of a donut comes out clean. Remove from the oven and allow to cool briefly in the pan before transferring to a wire rack to cool completely. Repeat with the remaining batter, if any.

If making the donuts in an electric donut maker, fill the bottom of the donut maker wells completely with batter, then close and secure the lid. Allow to bake for 3 minutes. Open the donut maker and remove the donuts with the remover tool included in the package or the tines of a fork or chocolate-dipping tool. Transfer to a wire rack to cool

---

2 cups (280 g) gluten-free cake flour (see page 2)

1½ teaspoons baking powder

¼ teaspoon baking soda

½ teaspoon kosher salt

¾ cup (150 g) granulated sugar

4 tablespoons (56 g) unsalted butter, at room temperature

1 egg (50 g, weighed out of shell) plus 1 egg white (25 g), at room temperature, beaten

¾ cup (6 fluid ounces) buttermilk, at room temperature

1 teaspoon pure vanilla extract

Confectioners' sugar, for coating

---

completely. Repeat with the remaining batter. Allow the donuts to cool briefly before dredging them through confectioners' sugar to coat.

The finished donuts can be stored in a sealed glass or plastic container at room temperature and should maintain their texture for at least 2 days. For longer storage, seal the finished donuts tightly in a freezer-safe wrap or bag, and freeze for up to 2 months. Defrost at room temperature. The sugar coating may shed a bit over time, but it won't affect the taste at all. The donuts can also be tossed in more confectioners' sugar before serving.

CHAPTER 6
I Want Candy!

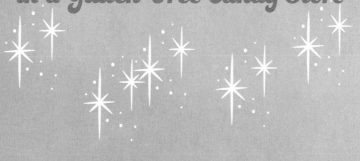

Like a Kid
in a Gluten-Free Candy Store

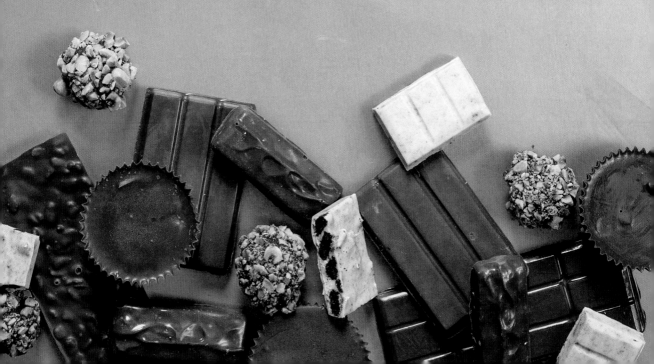

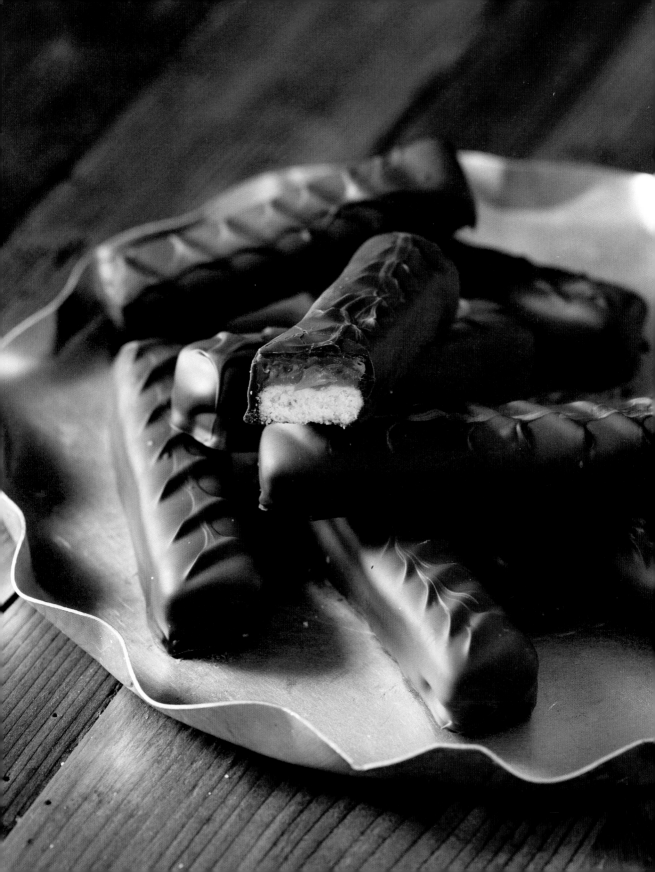

Mars Twix Caramel Cookie Bars

MAKES ABOUT 20 CANDY BARS

These rich milk chocolate candy bars with buttery short-bread and sweet soft caramel inside are just like you remember them to be. The easiest way to make the long, thin shortbread cookies for these bars is also the way they'll look and taste most authentic. The cookie dough is very easy to roll out and slice before baking, and the same holds true for cutting the soft caramel to size. Then, all that's left is a dip in plenty of milk chocolate topping and you will be flat-out amazed at how these really do taste like the packaged candy. The Soft Caramel for Candies (page 291) can be made at least a couple of weeks ahead of time and stored well sealed in plastic wrap at room temperature. And if you're hesitant to make your own soft caramel, you can purchase ready-made soft caramel from Chocoley.com (see Resources, page 295).

Prepare the cookies: Preheat your oven to 325°F. Line rimmed baking sheets with unbleached parchment paper and set them aside.

In a large bowl, place the cake flour, salt, and sugar, and whisk to combine well. Create a well in the center of the dry ingredients, add the butter and 1 tablespoon of the water, and knead until the dough comes together, using more water by the teaspoon if necessary. Place the dough between two sheets of unbleached parchment paper and roll into a rectangle about ½ inch thick. With a sharp knife or pizza or pastry wheel, slice into rectangles 3½ inches long and ½ inch wide. Place the rectangles 1 inch apart from one another on the prepared baking sheets. Using a toothpick or wooden skewer, press three holes, evenly spaced apart and each about ⅛ inch deep, into the top of each dough rectangle. Place the baking sheets in the center of the preheated oven and bake for about 10 minutes, or until just beginning to brown on the edges. Remove from the oven and allow to cool completely on the baking sheets.

Shortbread Cookie

1¾ cups (245 g) gluten-free cake flour (see page 2)

⅛ teaspoon kosher salt

½ cup (100 g) granulated sugar

8 tablespoons (112 g) unsalted butter, at room temperature

1 to 2 tablespoons (½ to 1 fluid ounce) lukewarm water

Caramel

Soft Caramel for Candies (page 291) or 1 pound premade soft caramel

Chocolate Topping

18 ounces milk chocolate, chopped

4 tablespoons (56 g) virgin coconut oil

Prepare the caramel: Roll out the caramel between two sheets of unbleached parchment paper into a rectangle about ½ inch thick. With a sharp knife or pizza or pastry wheel, cut the caramel into 3½ x ½-inch rectangles (the same size as the shortbread cookies). Place one caramel rectangle on top of each cooled shortbread cookie, and press gently to adhere.

Prepare the topping: Place the chocolate and coconut oil in a large, heat-safe bowl and melting according to the instructions on page 21. Allow the chocolate to sit at room temperature until it begins to thicken a bit. Immerse the caramel-topped shortbread, one at a time, in the glaze: Press down on it with the tines of a fork, then flip it gently in the chocolate. Pull the bar out of the chocolate by slipping the fork under it and bobbing it on the surface of the chocolate a few times before pulling it along the edge of the bowl and carefully placing it on a clean sheet of waxed or parchment paper. Allow the chocolate glaze to set at room temperature.

Once finished, the candy bars can be wrapped individually in plastic wrap and stored at cool room temperature for at least 5 days. For longer storage, wrap tightly in a freezer-safe bag, and freeze for up to 2 months. Defrost at room temperature.

Hershey's Kit Kat Crisp Wafers in Milk Chocolate

MAKES 8 BARS (3 "FINGERS" EACH)

Before you even ask me which is my "favorite" recipe in the book (what—you weren't going to ask?) let me tell you straight up that this recipe for Kit Kats is my crowning achievement. Tort wafers, the ridged wafers that come in sheets, can be difficult for a home baker to come by even in their gluten-containing form, and no one sells them gluten-free. After four years of recipe testing, I am happy to report that, not only are the lightly sweet wafers easy to make (just roll out the simple dough, bake it, score it into the proper small rectangles right out of the oven, and separate the individual wafers once cool), they even stay crisp and snappy when they're covered in layer upon layer of gorgeous milk chocolate. In fact, the wafers themselves are so good that I often keep a small glass jar of them in the kitchen for a light after-dinner snack. Cover them in chocolate, and you have yourself a gluten-free Kit Kat. It's a gluten-free culinary home run!

NOTE: For authentic candies, you'll need two Kit Kat–style chocolate mold sets (4 molds per set, 8 in total). (See Resources, page 294, for where to purchase.)

First, prepare the wafers: Preheat your oven to 325°F. In the bowl of a stand mixer fitted with the paddle attachment, or a large bowl and a hand mixer, beat the butter until light and fluffy. Add the sugar and vanilla, and beat until well combined. In a small bowl, place the flour, baking powder, and salt, and whisk to combine well. Add the dry ingredients to the creamed butter and sugar mixture in two batches, alternating with the 3 tablespoons of water and beginning and ending with the dry ingredients. The dough will come together and should be thick but

Crisp Wafers

5 tablespoons (70 g) unsalted butter, at room temperature

½ cup plus 2 tablespoons (125 g) granulated sugar

1 teaspoon pure vanilla extract

1 cup (140 g) all-purpose gluten-free flour (see page 2), plus more for sprinkling

½ teaspoon baking powder

¼ teaspoon kosher salt

3 tablespoons (1½ fluid ounces) lukewarm water, plus more if necessary

Candy Bars

18 ounces milk chocolate, chopped

4 tablespoons (56 g) virgin coconut oil

Crisp Wafers

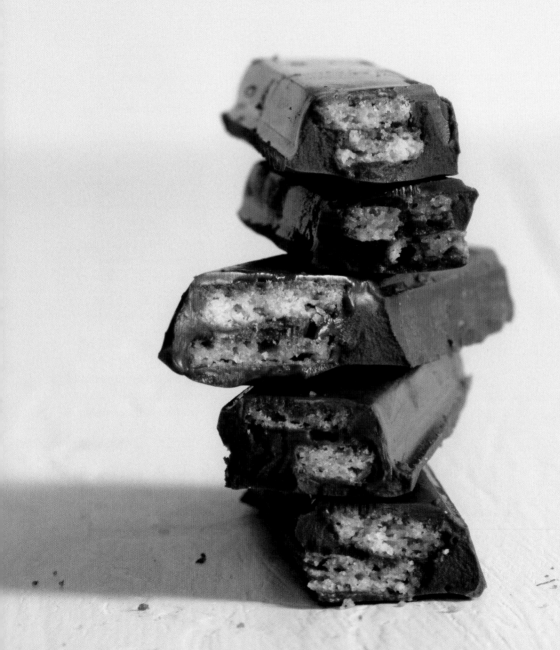

should not be stiff. If it is stiff, add more water by the half-teaspoonful as necessary and mix to combine.

Divide the dough in half, and place one piece on a large sheet of unbleached parchment paper. Pat it into a thick rectangle. Dust lightly with all-purpose flour and roll the dough into a 12 x 15-inch rectangle, a bit more than $\frac{1}{8}$ inch thick (no thinner), sprinkling lightly with flour as necessary to prevent sticking. Square the edges of the dough as best you can. Place the rectangle of dough, still on the parchment paper, flat on a half sheet pan. Have a sharp knife, pizza wheel or pastry wheel ready to score the dough as soon as it is baked. Place the dough in the center of the preheated oven and bake until very pale golden all over, about 12 minutes. Remove from the oven, and immediately score into smaller rectangles of about $\frac{1}{2}$ inch wide x 3 inches long. Allow to cool completely, and break the cooled wafers along the scoring. Repeat with the other piece of dough.

Assemble the candy bars: Place the chocolate and coconut oil in a medium-size, heat-safe bowl and melt according to the instructions on page 21. To make the candy, you will need 6 rectangular wafers per 3-finger candy bar. In each finger of a Kit Kat mold, pour a thin layer of melted milk chocolate in the bottom of each well. Layer one rectangular wafer on top of the chocolate. Cover with another layer of melted chocolate, followed by another wafer. Finish with a thick layer of chocolate to the top of the mold. Shake the mold gently back and forth to distribute the chocolate evenly without shifting the wafers around. Allow the chocolate to set completely in the molds before popping out the candy.

As mentioned earlier, the prepared crisp wafers will stay crisp in a sealed glass container for at least a week. Once finished, the candy bars can be wrapped individually in plastic wrap and stored at cool room temperature for at least 5 days. For longer storage, wrap tightly in a freezer-safe bag, and freeze for up to 2 months. Defrost at room temperature.

Hershey's Cookies 'n' Creme Candy Bars

MAKES 6 CHOCOLATE BARS

18 ounces white chocolate, chopped

1½ tablespoons (21 g) virgin coconut oil

8 ounces Nabisco Oreo Sandwich Cookies, Chocolate (page 53) or store-bought gluten-free chocolate creme sandwich cookies, crushed

*J*t's not like you couldn't have thought of this yourself. I get that. But did you really consider actually doing it until I reminded you just now of how much you miss cookies 'n' cream candy bars? K-Toos is a good brand of packaged gluten-free chocolate sandwich cookies, but they're crazy expensive. Trader Joe's also sells its own gluten-free variety of chocolate sandwich cookies called Gluten Free Joe-Joe's Chocolate Vanilla Cream Cookies, but the only cookies that really taste *just like Oreos* are what you see on page 53 of this very book.

NOTE: You will need two chocolate bar mold sets (each mold about 5 ½ inches across, 6 in total) (see page 295 for where to purchase) for this recipe.

In a medium-size, heat-safe bowl, place the chocolate and coconut oil, and melt according to the instructions on page 21. Add the crushed cookies and mix gently to combine. Pour the chocolate and cookie mixture into the molds, and shake back and forth into an even layer. Allow to set at room temperature.

Once finished, the candy bars can be wrapped individually in plastic wrap and stored at cool room temperature for at least 5 days. For longer storage, wrap tightly in a freezer-safe bag, and freeze for up to 2 months. Defrost at room temperature.

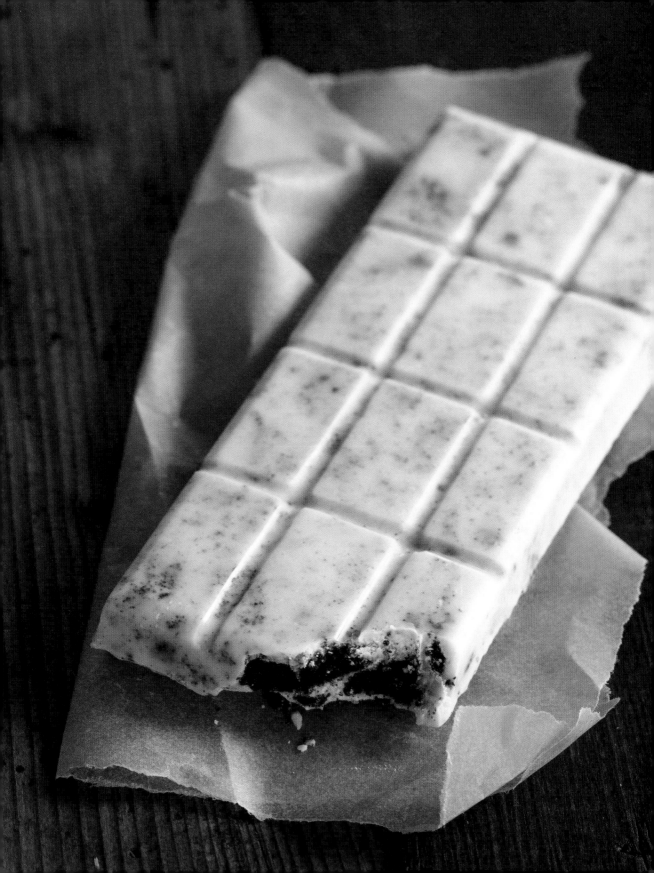

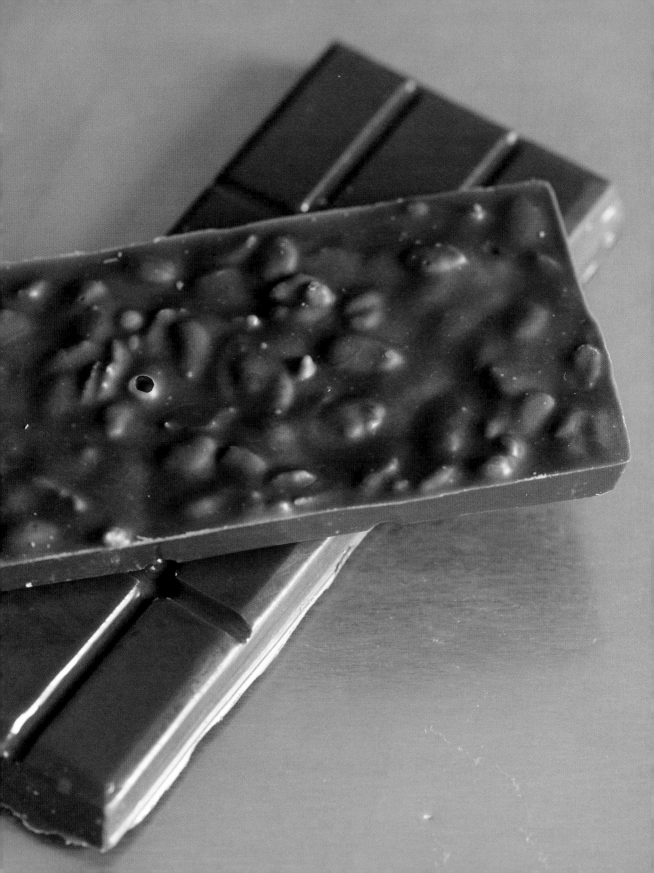

Nestlé Crunch Bars

MAKES 6 CHOCOLATE BARS

When you think of "crisp rice cereal," you probably think of Kellogg's Rice Krispies. Because Kellogg's also make a gluten-free version, you'd think that would be the best gluten-free crisp rice cereal. I bet you know where I'm going with this . . . Kellogg's Gluten-Free Rice Krispies cereal is adequate, but Erewhon Crispy Brown Rice Cereal (the kind with salt!) is much less bland and even a little crispier.

NOTE: *You will need two chocolate bar mold sets (each mold about 5½ inches across, 6 molds in total) (see page 295 for where to purchase) for this recipe.*

In a medium-size, heat-safe bowl, place the chocolate and coconut oil, and melt according to the instructions on page 21. Allow to cool until no longer hot to the touch. Add the rice cereal and mix gently to combine. If you add the rice cereal while the chocolate mixture is still hot, the cereal tends to taste as if it has become stale. Pour the chocolate and rice cereal into the molds, and shake back and forth into an even layer. Allow to set at room temperature.

Once finished, the candy bars can be wrapped individually in plastic wrap and stored at cool room temperature for at least 5 days. For longer storage, wrap tightly in a freezer-safe bag, and freeze for up to 2 months. Defrost at room temperature.

---

18 ounces milk chocolate, chopped

1½ tablespoons (21 g) virgin coconut oil

2 cups (60 g) gluten-free crisp rice cereal

Nestlé 100 Grand Chocolate Bars

MAKES 12 BARS

Soft Caramel for Candies
(page 291) or 1 pound
premade soft caramel

24 ounces milk chocolate,
chopped

5 tablespoons (70 g)
virgin coconut oil

2 cups (60 g) gluten-free
crisp rice cereal

Nestlé's 100 Grand Chocolate Bars are the sort of candy bar that is easily made gluten-free—just use your favorite gluten-free crisp rice cereal and get to work. Once you make the Soft Caramel for Candies (page 291) and cut it to size, these candy bars practically make themselves. To make things even easier, purchase premade soft caramel from Chocoley.com (see Resources, page 295). It's very shelf-stable and easy to work with. If you don't want to use the special candy molds, just freestyle it by lining up the pieces of caramel and pouring the chocolate-crisp rice mixture over the top.

NOTE: As noted above, for tidy chocolate bars, you'll need two small chocolate candy molds (each bar about 3 x 1 x ¾-inch) (see page 295 for where to purchase).

Place the soft caramel between two pieces of unbleached parchment paper and roll out into a rectangle about ½ inch thick. Remove the top piece of parchment paper, and, using a very sharp knife or pizza or pastry wheel, slice 12 pieces of caramel, each 3 inches long x 1 inch wide (and ½ inch high). Set the caramel pieces aside.

Place the chocolate and coconut oil in a large heat-safe bowl and melt according to the instructions on page 21. Allow to cool until no longer hot to the touch. Add the rice cereal and stir gently to combine.

In each chocolate candy mold, place a thin layer of the chocolate crispy mixture, then place the soft caramel rectangle and press the caramel down a bit. Top with enough of the chocolate crispy mixture fill the rest of the mold to the top. Shake the mold gently back and forth to distribute the chocolate evenly in the mold. Allow the chocolate to set completely in the molds before popping out the candy.

Once finished, the candy bars can be wrapped individually in plastic wrap and stored at cool room temperature for at least 5 days. For longer storage, wrap tightly in a freezer-safe bag, and freeze for up to 2 months. Defrost at room temperature.

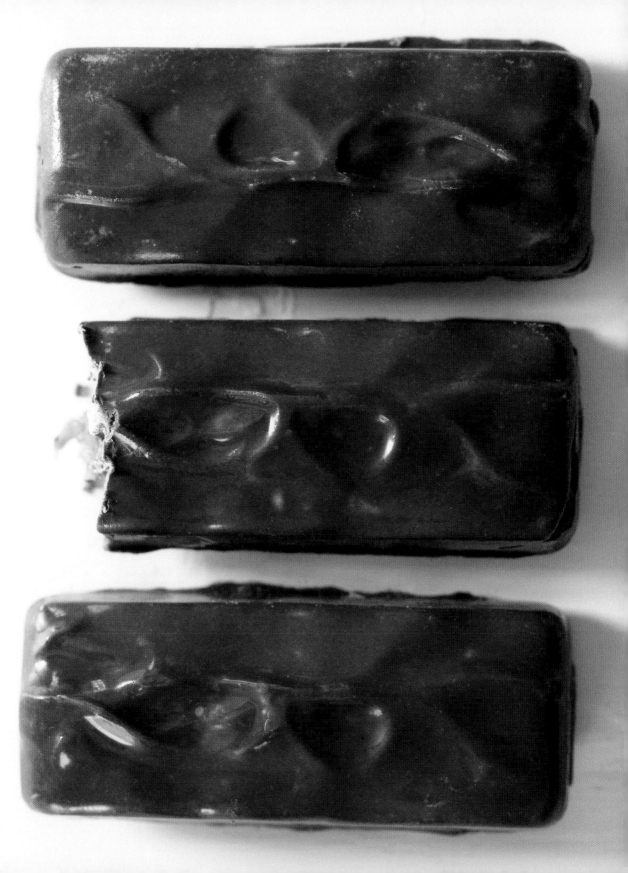

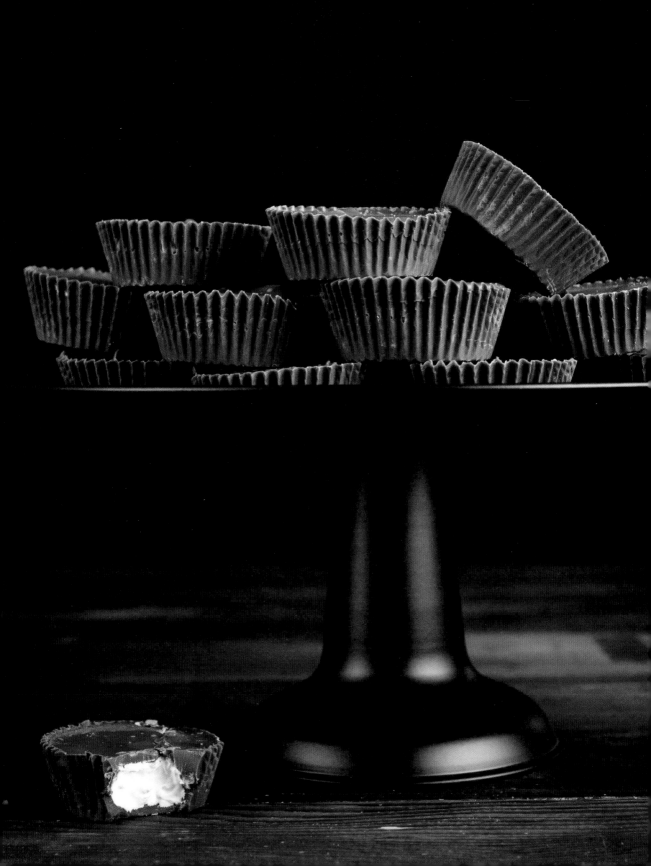

Boyer Mallo Cups

MAKES 12 CUPS

Near as I can tell, the original Boyer Mallo Cups are . . . naturally gluten-free. So why am I including a recipe for them in this cookbook? You mean, other than the fact that the photo is absolutely stunning and I'm considering wallpapering my kitchen with it? Because these are *gasp* even better than the original. The goal of most of the recipes in this book is to make a dead ringer for the original snack or dessert. But sometimes, we can do even better. This is one of those times. Plus, you can make it with dark chocolate instead of milk chocolate and practically call it health food with a straight face.

¾ cup (60 g) coconut flakes

24 ounces milk chocolate, chopped

6 tablespoons (84 g) virgin coconut oil

1 recipe Marshmallow Fluff (page 166)

Line a standard twelve-cup muffin tin with muffin liners and set it aside. Preheat your oven to 275°F.

Line a rimmed baking sheet with unbleached parchment paper, and scatter the coconut flakes on the baking sheet in a single layer. Place in the center of the preheated oven and bake until the coconut is fragrant and beginning to brown around the edges, about 7 minutes, taking care not to let them burn. Remove from the oven and allow to cool on the baking sheet before crushing with your hands into smaller pieces.

Prepare the Marshmallow Fluff: In a medium-size, heat-safe bowl, place the chocolate and coconut oil, and melt according to the instructions on page 21. Using a large, spring-loaded ice-cream scoop, place 1½ to 2 tablespoons of melted chocolate in the bottom of each muffin liner. Working quickly before the chocolate begins to set, divide about half of the crushed toasted coconut chips among the wells, and press gently into the chocolate with a spoon to immerse the coconut in the chocolate and force the chocolate up the sides of the liners a bit. Clean the ice-cream scoop and then use it to place about 1½ tablespoons of Marshmallow Fluff on top of the coconut in the center of each cup, sprinkle with the remaining crushed toasted coconut, and top with another 2 tablespoons of melted chocolate. Shake the muffin tin back and forth and side to side to distribute the chocolate evenly in each muffin liner. Allow to set at room temperature.

Once finished, the cups can be wrapped individually in plastic wrap and stored at cool room temperature for at least 5 days. For longer storage, wrap tightly in a freezer-safe bag, and freeze for up to 2 months. Defrost at room temperature or you'll nearly crack your teeth trying to bite into them!

Ferrero Rocher Fine Hazelnut Chocolates

MAKES ABOUT 30 CANDIES

Making the truffles for these fancy little chocolate hazelnut candies takes a few steps, but it's easy to make the candies in stages. The crunchy hazelnut wafer cookies can even be made a couple weeks ahead of time and crushed into crumbs right away, then stored in a sealed glass container at room temperature. Storing them in glass will keep the crumbs from getting soggy. Luckily, Nutella, at least as sold in the United States, is gluten-free, so there's no need to make our own hazelnut spread for use in the candy truffles. I like to buy hazelnut flour at Nuts.com. You can also buy raw shelled hazelnuts and toast them as explained below. Then, instead of chopping the skinned nuts, simply process them in a food processor with a teaspoon of cornstarch or potato starch just until you have a powder. The starch will help prevent the nuts from being processed into a nut butter.

First, prepare the wafer cookies: Preheat your oven to 325°F. Line a rimmed baking sheet with unbleached parchment paper and set it aside.

In a large bowl, place the flour, cornstarch, hazelnut flour, baking soda, salt, and sugar, and whisk to combine well. Create a well in the center of the dry ingredients and add the butter, egg whites, and vanilla, and mix to combine. The dough will be thick. Divide the dough into small pieces, about 1 tablespoonful each. Roll each into a ball, press into a disk about 1/8 inch thick and place on the prepared baking sheet about 1 inch apart from one another.

Place in the center of the preheated oven and bake until lightly golden brown around the edges and firm to the touch, about 10 minutes. Remove from the oven and allow to cool on the baking sheet for 10 minutes before transferring to a wire rack to cool completely. Once

Hazelnut Wafer Cookies

(MAKES 24 COOKIES)

1½ cups (210 g) all-purpose gluten-free flour (see page 2)

¼ cup (36 g) cornstarch

½ cup (60 g) hazelnut flour (see headnote)

½ teaspoon baking soda

⅛ teaspoon kosher salt

¼ cup (50 g) granulated sugar

8 tablespoons (112 g) unsalted butter, at room temperature

2 egg whites (50 g), at room temperature

1 teaspoon pure vanilla extract

CONTINUED ON PAGE 283

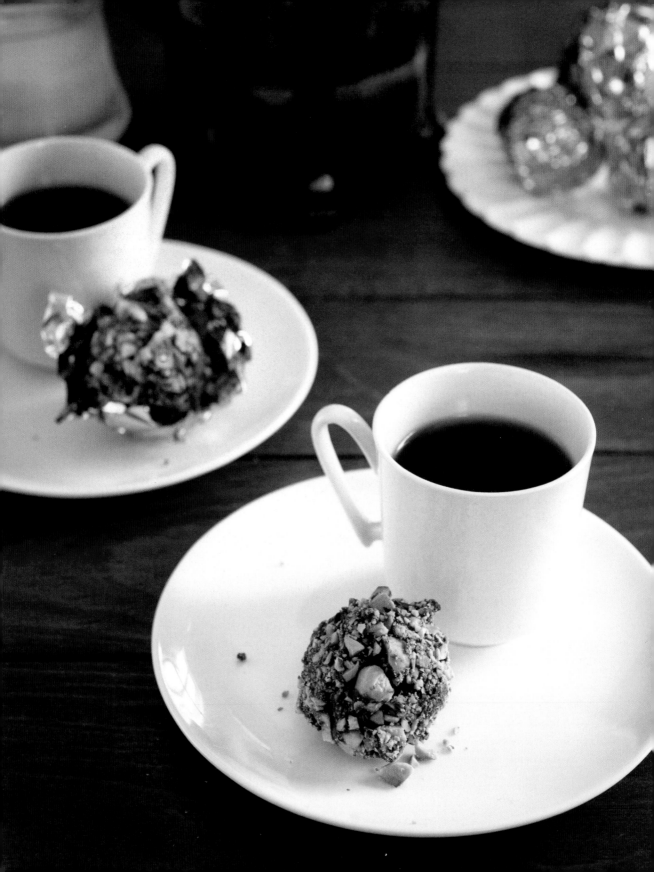

cool, with the heel of your hand on a flat surface, crush the cookies into small crumbs.

Toast the raw shelled hazelnuts listed for both the candy truffles and chocolate coating (a total of 1⅓ cups [180 g]). Reduce the oven temperature to 250°F and line a rimmed baking sheet with unbleached parchment paper. Place the whole shelled nuts in an even layer on the prepared baking sheet. Place them in the preheated oven for about 15 minutes, or until fragrant. Remove from the oven and transfer the warm toasted nuts to a clean tea towel. Wrap the nuts up in the towel and allow them to steam for a few minutes. This will help the skins on the nuts come off easily. Rub the towel on the nuts to remove as many of the skins as possible. Roughly chop the nuts and set them aside.

Prepare the candy truffles: Place all the truffle ingredients (measure out ⅔ cup of the toasted hazelnuts) in a large bowl and mix together until smooth. Cover the bowl with plastic wrap and chill until the mixture can be shaped into balls. Line a rimmed baking sheet with unbleached parchment paper and set it aside. Remove the truffle mixture from the refrigerator and roll it tightly into balls, each about 1 inch in diameter. Place the truffles on the prepared baking sheet and place in the refrigerator to chill until firm.

Prepare the coating: Line a rimmed baking sheet with parchment or waxed paper and set it aside. Place the chocolate and coconut oil in a medium-size, heat-safe bowl and melt according to the instructions on page 21. Immerse each truffle in the chocolate mixture, press down on the truffle with a dipping tool or fork, flip it over in the chocolate, remove the truffle with the utensil, and place on the prepared baking sheet. Sprinkle each chocolate-covered truffle with the remaining ⅔ cup chopped, toasted hazelnuts and gently press the nuts to the chocolate so they adhere. Allow to set at room temperature.

Once finished, the candies can be wrapped individually and stored at cool room temperature for at least 5 days. For longer storage, wrap tightly in a freezer-safe bag, and freeze for up to 2 months. Defrost at room temperature.

CONTINUED FROM PAGE 281

Candy Truffles

1 recipe Hazelnut Wafer Cookies, crushed into small crumbs (about 2 cups crumbs)

⅔ cup (90 g) raw shelled hazelnuts

½ cup (150 g) Nutella hazelnut spread

Chocolate Coating

12 ounces dark chocolate, chopped

3 tablespoons (42 g) virgin coconut oil

⅔ cup (90 g) raw shelled hazelnuts

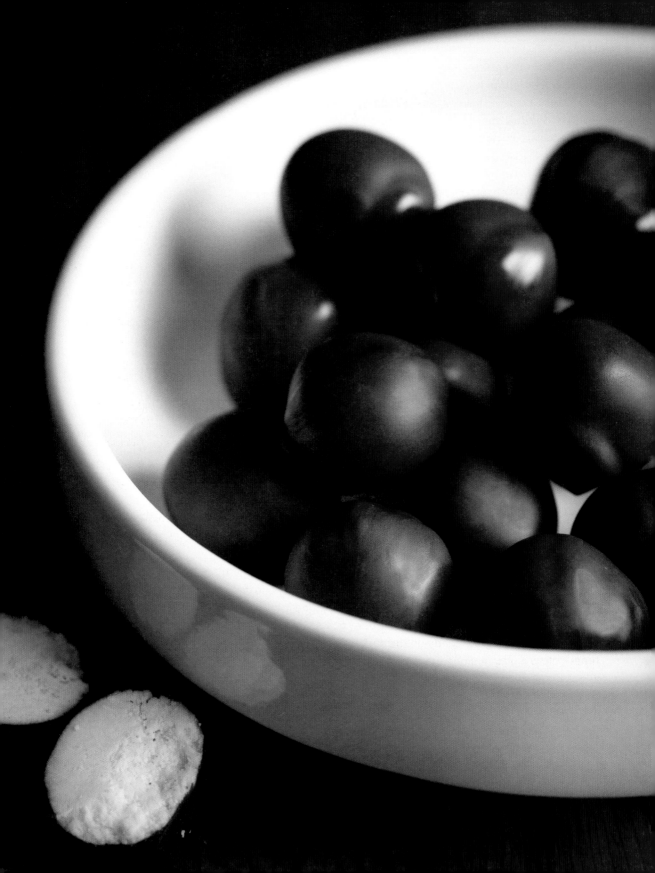

Whoppers Original Malted Milk Balls

MAKES ABOUT 35 CANDIES

*C*learly, these chocolate-covered crunchy-soft milk candies are *not* malted. Malt is derived from barley, one of the "big three" gluten-containing grains (wheat-barley-rye). But that doesn't mean that we can't approximate the rich malty taste and smooth but crunchy texture of Whoppers. It just takes the right mix of basic ingredients. And, of course, we cover them in rich milk chocolate.

First, prepare the candies: Line a large rimmed baking sheet with unbleached parchment paper and set it aside.

In a large, heat-safe bowl, melt the white chocolate as instructed on page 21. Add the remaining white chocolate candy ingredients (except for the water) and mix everything together. If the mixture doesn't hold together, add water by the half-teaspoonful until small pieces hold together well when squeezed in the palm of your hand. Shape the mixture into tightly packed 1-inch balls, adding more water as necessary. Place the candies about ½ inch apart from one another on the prepared baking sheet, and allow to sit at room temperature for 10 to 12 hours, until dry and firm. (It does take that long!)

Once the candies are firm, prepare the topping: Place the milk chocolate and coconut oil in a large, heat-safe bowl and melt according to the instructions on page 21. Immerse each piece of candy in the chocolate mixture: Press down on it with a dipping tool or fork, flip it over in the chocolate, and remove the candy with the utensil by slipping the utensil under it and bobbing the candy on the surface of the chocolate a few times before pulling it along the edge of the bowl. Place on a piece of waxed or parchment paper.

Once finished, the candies can be stored in a sealed glass container and stored at cool room temperature for at least 3 to 5 days, after which the candies may lose their crunchiness, but will still be delicious. They do not maintain their texture during freezing.

White Chocolate Candies

6 ounces white chocolate, chopped

5 tablespoons (30 g) nonfat dry milk, ground into a fine powder

2 tablespoons (18 g) cornstarch

1 teaspoon pure vanilla extract

⅛ teaspoon kosher salt

Water by the half-teaspoonful, as necessary

Chocolate Topping

12 ounces milk chocolate, chopped

3 tablespoons (42 g) virgin coconut oil

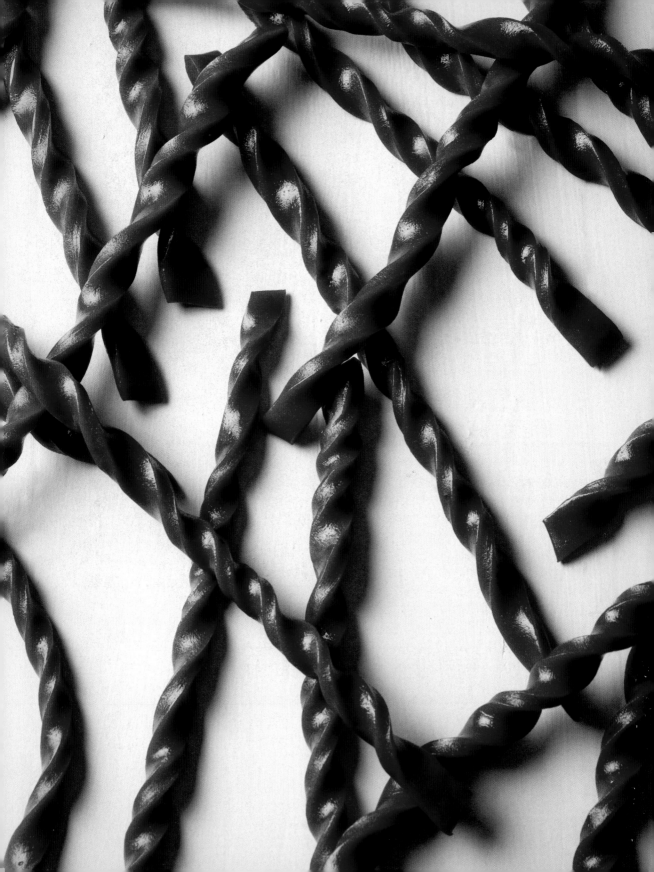

Red Cherry Licorice

MAKES ABOUT 24 PIECES, DEPENDING UPON SIZE

*F*ile licorice under the category of candies that most people would assume are naturally gluten-free, but simply . . . aren't, as they're traditionally wheat-based. These are not exactly like Twizzlers; to me, Twizzlers (although delicious) are more about texture than flavor. This licorice is more like a cross between Twizzlers and truly flavorful Red Vines licorice. It's sweet and smooth, with authentic-tasting cherry flavoring, as LorAnn flavoring oils are quite true to taste. If you are able to find Lyle's golden syrup, use that, not honey, as honey has its own distinct flavor that tends to compete with the cherry flavor. This recipe will go smoothly if you work quickly, so having all the ingredients prepared and in place near the stovetop will go a long way—and don't forget your candy thermometer! If your sugar mixture doesn't reach the proper temperature, the licorice will not set up.

Grease and line with unbleached parchment paper a 9-inch square baking dish and set it aside. In a small bowl, place the flour and salt, and whisk to combine well. Set the remaining ingredients to the side within arm's reach of the stovetop.

In a large, heavy-bottomed saucepan, place the butter, sugar, corn syrup, condensed milk, and golden syrup. Clip a candy thermometer to the side of the saucepan and cook over medium-high heat until the mixture reaches a boil, stirring constantly. Lower the heat to medium so the mixture maintains a slow boil, and continue to cook until the temperature reaches 240°F.

Remove the mixture from the heat and add all the flour mixture to the cooked sugar mixture. Working quickly, mix well, and add the cherry flavoring oil and food coloring (I use a toothpick to add gel food

½ cup (70 g) all-purpose gluten-free flour (see page 2)

¼ teaspoon kosher salt

8 tablespoons (112 g) unsalted butter, at room temperature

1 cup (200 g) granulated sugar

½ cup (168 g) light corn syrup

½ cup (156 g) sweetened condensed milk

4 tablespoons (84 g) Lyle's golden syrup or honey

½ teaspoon cherry flavoring oil (LorAnn brand is gluten-free)

About ¼ teaspoon red gel food coloring, or as desired (AmeriColor brand is gluten-free)

coloring a bit at a time, as specific measurements are not essential). Mix well again.

Pour the candy into the prepared baking dish, and shake it back and forth so that it is in an even layer. Place the baking dish in the refrigerator to chill for 30 minutes. Remove the baking dish from the refrigerator, and lift up on the parchment paper to remove the candy in one piece from the baking dish. Place on a flat surface. With kitchen shears or a pastry or pizza wheel, cut the square of candy in half, and then cut each half into ¼-inch-wide strips. Twist the strips at both ends to create the traditional licorice spiral. Allow to sit at room temperature until slightly hardened, and serve.

These can be stored in a single layer in a sealed glass or plastic container and stored at cool room temperature for at least 5 days. For longer storage, place the container in the refrigerator for up to 2 weeks, and allow to come to room temperature before eating.

Black Licorice

Black licorice separates the whole world into two camps: those who love it and those who hate it. If you're a lover, you're in luck! You can now make your own, and it's sure to have that true anise flavor with LorAnn flavoring oil. Plus, you can even replace the Lyle's golden syrup or honey with molasses, something you can't do with the Red Cherry Licorice (page 287) because no one wants red licorice with unsightly dark flecks from dark-colored molasses. In fact, if you do use molasses and you're not particularly concerned with achieving a true black color in your black licorice, feel free to skip the food coloring altogether. As with the red cherry licorice, be sure to begin by assembling all of your ingredients, plus your candy thermometer, near the stovetop so you can move quickly and nimbly.

½ cup (70 g) all-purpose gluten-free flour (see page 2)

¼ teaspoon kosher salt

8 tablespoons (112 g) unsalted butter, at room temperature

1 cup (200 g) granulated sugar

½ cup (168 g) light corn syrup

½ cup (156 g) sweetened condensed milk

4 tablespoons (84 g) Lyle's golden syrup or honey

½ teaspoon anise flavoring oil (LorAnn brand is gluten-free)

About ¼ teaspoon black gel food coloring, or as desired (AmeriColor brand is gluten-free)

Grease and line with unbleached parchment paper a 9-inch square baking dish and set it aside. In a small bowl, place the flour and salt, and whisk to combine well. Set the remaining ingredients to the side within arm's reach of the stovetop.

In a large, heavy-bottomed saucepan, place the butter, sugar, corn syrup, condensed milk, and golden syrup. Clip a candy thermometer to the side of the saucepan and cook over medium-high heat until the mixture reaches a boil, stirring constantly. Lower the heat to medium so the mixture maintains a slow boil, and continue to cook until the temperature reaches 240°F.

Remove the mixture from the heat and add all the flour mixture to the cooked sugar mixture. Working quickly, mix well, and add the anise flavoring oil and black food coloring (I use a toothpick to add gel food coloring a bit at a time, as specific measurements are not essential). Mix well again.

Pour the candy into the prepared baking dish, and shake it back and forth so that it is in an even layer. Place the baking dish in the refrigerator to chill for 30 minutes. Remove the baking dish from the refrigerator, and lift up on the parchment paper to remove the candy in one piece from the baking dish. Place on a flat surface. With kitchen shears or a pastry or pizza wheel, cut the square of candy in half, and then cut each half into ¼-inch-wide strips. Twist the strips at both ends to create the traditional licorice spiral. Allow to sit at room temperature until slightly hardened, and serve.

These can be stored in a single layer in a sealed glass or plastic container and stored at cool room temperature for at least 5 days. For longer storage, place the container in the refrigerator for up to 2 weeks, and allow to come to room temperature before eating.

Soft Caramel for Candies

MAKES ABOUT 1 POUND CARAMEL

If you just.don't want.to.make.caramel at home (even though I promise it's so easy!), you can buy ready-made soft caramel online at Chocoley.com, a great resource for all things related to home chocolate candy–making (see Resources, page 295). Chocoley's soft caramel comes in a tub, and although it isn't cheap, it can be used for every recipe in this book that calls for "Soft Caramel for Candies." I don't recommend using Kraft soft caramel candies as they are too soft for the recipes in this book. This recipe will teach you how to make your own soft caramel, though, and I think it's worth it. A tip when cooking sugar: Slow and steady wins the race. If you raise the heat under the saucepan to speed up the cooking time, the caramel is likely to burn. And be sure to use your candy thermometer, paying careful attention to it as the temperature climbs. This caramel will keep quite well at room temperature for at least two weeks when wrapped tightly, as the high sugar content acts as a natural preservative. If it begins to harden, you can microwave the portion you intend to use at 50% power for ten seconds at a time until it is softened enough to shape.

2 cups (400 g) granulated sugar

½ cup (4 fluid ounces) water

¼ teaspoon cream of tartar

¾ cup (6 fluid ounces) heavy whipping cream

5 tablespoons (70 g) unsalted butter, chopped

1 teaspoon pure vanilla extract

Line a quarter sheet (13 x 9 x 1-inch) pan with unbleached parchment paper and set it aside.

In a medium-size, heavy-bottomed saucepan, place the sugar, water, and cream of tartar and whisk to combine. Clip a candy thermometer to the side of the saucepan and cook, undisturbed, over medium-high heat until the sugar begins to turn amber-colored around the edges and reaches 300°F. Remove the saucepan from the heat, stir to prevent the sugar from burning, and add the cream. The mixture will bubble up quite a lot. Stir until the bubbling subsides. The sugar may seize up, but it will melt again. Add the butter, and stir to combine. Return the saucepan to the heat and cook, undisturbed, over medium-high heat until the mixture reaches 245°F. Remove from the heat and whisk in the vanilla.

Pour the hot caramel into the prepared pan (without scraping the bottom of the saucepan) and shake it back and forth and side to side into an even layer. Allow to sit at room temperature until set, at least 2 hours. Once cool, the caramel can be covered in plastic and stored in a cool, dry place for up to a month.

Metric Conversions

The recipes in this book have not been tested with metric measurements, so some variations might occur. Remember that the weight of dry ingredients varies according to the volume or density factor: 1 cup of flour weighs far less than 1 cup of sugar, and 1 tablespoon doesn't necessarily hold 3 teaspoons.

GENERAL FORMULA FOR METRIC CONVERSION

Ounces to grams	multiply ounces by 28.35
Grams to ounces	multiply grams by 0.035
Pounds to grams	multiply pounds by 453.5
Pounds to kilograms	multiply pounds by 0.45
Cups to liters	multiply cups by 0.24
Fahrenheit to Celsius	subtract 32 from Fahrenheit temperature, multiply by 5, divide by 9
Celsius to Fahrenheit	multiply Celsius temperature by 9, divide by 5, add 32

VOLUME (LIQUID) MEASUREMENTS

1 teaspoon	= $\frac{1}{6}$ fluid ounce	= 5 milliliters
1 tablespoon	= $\frac{1}{2}$ fluid ounce	= 15 milliliters
2 tablespoons	= 1 fluid ounce	= 30 milliliters
$\frac{1}{4}$ cup	= 2 fluid ounces	= 60 milliliters
$\frac{1}{3}$ cup	= $2\frac{2}{3}$ fluid ounces	= 79 milliliters
$\frac{1}{2}$ cup	= 4 fluid ounces	= 118 milliliters
1 cup or $\frac{1}{2}$ pint	= 8 fluid ounces	= 250 milliliters
2 cups or 1 pint	= 16 fluid ounces	= 500 milliliters
4 cups or 1 quart	= 32 fluid ounces	= 1,000 milliliters
1 gallon	= 4 liters	

WEIGHT (MASS) MEASUREMENTS

1 ounce	= 30 grams	
2 ounces	= 55 grams	
3 ounces	= 85 grams	
4 ounces	= $\frac{1}{4}$ pound	= 125 grams
8 ounces	= $\frac{1}{2}$ pound	= 240 grams
12 ounces	= $\frac{3}{4}$ pound	= 375 grams
16 ounces	= 1 pound	= 454 grams

OVEN TEMPERATURE EQUIVALENTS, FAHRENHEIT (F) AND CELSIUS (C)

100°F	= 38°C
200°F	= 95°C
250°F	= 120°C
300°F	= 150°C
350°F	= 180°C
400°F	= 205°C
450°F	= 230°C

VOLUME (DRY) MEASUREMENTS

$\frac{1}{4}$ teaspoon	= 1 milliliter
$\frac{1}{2}$ teaspoon	= 2 milliliters
$\frac{3}{4}$ teaspoon	= 4 milliliters
1 teaspoon	= 5 milliliters
1 tablespoon	= 15 milliliters
$\frac{1}{4}$ cup	= 59 milliliters
$\frac{1}{3}$ cup	= 79 milliliters
$\frac{1}{2}$ cup	= 118 milliliters
$\frac{2}{3}$ cup	= 158 milliliters
$\frac{3}{4}$ cup	= 177 milliliters
1 cup	= 225 milliliters
4 cups or 1 quart	= 1 liter
$\frac{1}{2}$ gallon	= 2 liters
1 gallon	= 4 liters

LINEAR MEASUREMENTS

$\frac{1}{2}$ inch	= 1$\frac{1}{2}$ cm
1 inch	= 2$\frac{1}{2}$ cm
6 inches	= 15 cm
8 inches	= 20 cm
10 inches	= 25 cm
12 inches	= 30 cm
20 inches	= 50 cm

Resources

AMAZON.COM: http://www.amazon.com. For everything from pastry tips, cookie cutters, and meringue powder to, well, a microwave, Amazon is a reliable source for so much. I have a number of Ateco brand cookie cutter sets (a set each of plain round cutters, fluted round cutters, small polygon shapes, and plain oval cutters), each of which comes in its own flat, covered tin, and I have found all of them at Amazon. I also have ordered the following products from Amazon: Pomona Pectin; Honeyville almond flour; If You Care brand unbleached parchment paper and mini and large baking cups; Nordic Ware stainless-steel half sheet (18 x 13 x 1-inch) and quarter sheet (13 x 9 x 1-inch) rimmed baking sheets as well as standard muffin and miniature muffin tins; a Nordic Ware Pocket Pie Crimper (for Hostess Apple Fruit Pies, page 135); a candy/deep-fry thermometer; AmeriColor gel food colorings; LorAnn Oil flavoring oils and meringue powder; Great Lakes unflavored powdered gelatin (both cold- and hot-soluble varieties); Ateco pastry tips; chocolate-dipping tools; Authentic Foods superfine rice flours; all the specialty Wilton cake pans used for Twinkies (page 129), Sno Balls (page 137), and Ring Dings (page 155); a Wilton miniature donut pan; and even some of the Fat Daddio brand specialty snack cake pans. The Hostess brand Twinkie pan (which I don't own) and the USA Pans cake panel pan (useful for Drake's Coffee Cakes, page 149, and VitaTops muffin tops, pages 239–246) are also available at Amazon.

AUTHENTIC FOODS: http://www.authenticfoods.com. For gluten-free superfine white and brown rice flours, Authentic Foods is the only brand I know that exists. You can shop online directly in the Authentic Foods marketplace at http://www.glutenfree-supermarket.com/, purchase online at Amazon.com (free shipping if you are an Amazon Prime member), or in certain select brick-and-mortar stores.

BED, BATH & BEYOND: http://www.bedbathandbeyond.com. Bed, Bath & Beyond (BB&B) has long been, and remains, a go-to source of kitchen supplies and equipment. I regularly receive 20 percent–off coupons in the mail, and every BB&B store I have ever shopped in has always happily accepted expired 20 percent–off coupons. I have bought half (18 x 13 x 1-inch) and quarter (13 x 9 x 1-inch) sheet pans, standard and miniature muffin tins, a French rolling pin, chocolate-dipping tools, Epicurean brand cutting boards (a favorite of mine), glass and plastic storage containers, a candy/deep-fry thermometer, oven thermometers, measuring cups and spoons, and many other items there. Bed, Bath & Beyond also sells many USA Pans brand specialty baking pans, such as the cake panel pan.

CHOCOLEY: http://www.chocoley.com. Chocoley is a great source for pretempered chocolates (one formula for dipping, another formula for molding), ready-made soft caramel for candies, plus chocolate and candy molds and supplies.

COPPERGIFTS.COM: http://www.coppergifts.com. The one and only source I have ever found, online or otherwise, for what I consider to be a proper Goldfish cracker (page 179) cutter is CopperGifts.com. It is the "mini fish cookie cutter" and can be found under "Aquatic Animal Cookie Cutters" on the site. I also purchased the 3-inch hexagon cookie cutter on this site that I use to make Little Debbie Zebra Cakes (page 121). Be advised, though: The cutters on CopperGifts.com are not cheap.

COUNTRY KITCHEN SWEETART: http://www.countrykitchensa.com. I have purchased a number of chocolate bar and bite-size candy and chocolate molds here. It is also a source for AmeriColor gel food coloring and LorAnn flavoring oils.

FANCY FLOURS: http://www.fancyflours.com. Fancy Flours is a great source for cookie cutters. For the animal cookie cutters I used in the Nabisco Barnum's Animal Crackers on page 200, search Fancy Flours for its set of four "cookie stamp and cutters zoo animals theme" cutters. Fancy Flours also sells AmeriColor gel food coloring.

FANTE'S: http://fantes.com. Fante's is a kitchen supply store in the Italian Market section of Philadelphia, Pennsylvania. It's a relatively small store, but it seems to carry everything under the sun in its category. They have many, many different sets of cookie cutters, including plain round and fluted round Ateco cutter sets, and the rectangular set that I use for the Nabisco Graham Crackers (see page 195), as well as the spring-loaded Birkmann Linzer Shortbread Cutter that I use for a number of the Keebler crackers in Chapter 4. Many, if not most, of the items that Fante's sells in its store are also available online at http://fantes.com/. Visit http://fantes.com/cookie-cutter-sets .html for a comprehensive list of the cookie cutters available.

GLOBAL SUGAR ART: http://www.globalsugarart.com/index.php. Global Sugar Art is another source for candy bar chocolate molds, Kit Kat–style chocolate molds, and chocolate bar molds. It is also a source for LorAnn flavoring oils and AmeriColor gel food colorings and powdered food coloring.

KOHL'S: http://www.kohls.com. You might not think of Kohl's discount department stores as kitchen supply stores, but I have found my local store to be a great source for kitchen supplies large and small. At Kohl's, I have purchased everything from open-stock heavy-bottomed saucepans and the best silicone spoonulas ever invented (the Food Network brand sold at Kohl's is the best!) to muffin tins and my Babycakes electric donut maker (a favorite very small appliance of mine). Kohl's is very coupon-friendly, and even if you do not receive its coupons in the mail, cashiers often have a coupon available at the checkout register.

NUTS.COM: http://www.nuts.com. For certified gluten-free varieties of dried and freeze-dried fruits and vegetables, good-quality tapioca flour/starch (not all are created equal!), potato starch, potato flour, xanthan gum, cornstarch, raw nuts and nut pieces of all kinds, nut flours, and miniature M&Ms and Sixlets, Nuts.com is a great resource. Its shipping costs are high, though, but you do better if you buy larger quantities and/or more product, so I try to order only when I have a substantial list.

SUR LA TABLE: http://www.surlatable.com. This kitchen supply store carries most of the basic kitchen equipment on pages 18–23, but it is listed here specifically as one of the sources for the Fat Daddio specialty snack cakes pans used in Chapter 3.

SWEET BAKING SUPPLY: http://www.sweetbakingsupply.com. This is another source of chocolate bar and Kit Kat–style chocolate molds. It is also a source for AmeriColor gel food coloring and LorAnn flavoring oils.

List of Trademarks

Archway Soft Iced Oatmeal Cookies
Babycakes Mini Donut Maker
Barney Butter
Better Batter Gluten Free All Purpose Flour Mix
Boyer Mallo Cups
Choco Creme Snack Cake Pan
Cup4Cup Gluten Free Flour
Do-Si-Dos Girl Scout Cookies (a.k.a. Peanut Butter Sandwiches)
Drake's Coffee Cakes
Drake's Devil Dogs
Drake's Ring Dings
Drake's Sunny Doodles
Drake's Yodels
Earth Balance Buttery Sticks
Entenmann's Little Bites Blueberry Muffins
Entenmann's Little Bites Brownies
Entenmann's Little Bites Chocolate Chip Muffins
Entenmann's Devil's Food Donuts
Fat Daddio Classic Chocolate-Covered Wheel Cupcake
Ferrero Rocher Fine Hazelnut Chocolates
Fiber One Chewy Bars, Oats and Chocolate
Fiber One Chewy Bars, Oats and Peanut Butter
Gluten Free Joe-Joe's Chocolate Vanilla Cream Cookies
Hershey's Cookies'n'Creme Candy Bars
Hershey's Kit Kat Crisp Wafers in Milk Chocolate
Hershey's Special Dark [cocoa powder]
Hostess Apple Fruit Pies
Hostess Chocolate Cupcakes
Hostess Ding Dongs
Hostess Ho-Hos
Hostess Powdered Sugar Donettes

Hostess Sno Balls
Hostess Twinkies
Keebler Club Crackers, Multi-Grain
Keebler Club Crackers, Original
Keebler Fudge Stripes Cookies, Original
Keebler Sandies Dark Chocolate Almond Shortbread Cookies
Keebler Sandies Pecan Shortbread Cookies
Keebler Simply Made Butter Cookies
Keebler Soft Batch Chocolate Chip Cookies
Keebler Town House Crackers, Original
Keebler Vienna Fingers Creme Filled Sandwich Cookies
Kellogg's Frosted Brown Sugar Cinnamon Pop-Tarts Toaster Pastries
Kellogg's Frosted Chocolate Fudge Pop-Tarts Toaster Pastries
Kellogg's Frosted Strawberry Pop-Tarts Toaster Pastries
Kellogg's Gone Nutty! Frosted Chocolate Peanut Butter Pop-Tarts Toaster Pastries
Kellogg's Nutri-Grain Cereal Bars Apple Cinnamon
Kellogg's Nutri-Grain Cereal Bars, Strawberry
Kellogg's Pop-Tarts
Lemonades Girl Scout Cookies
Little Debbie Cosmic Brownies
Little Debbie Fudge Rounds
Little Debbie Oatmeal Creme Pies
Little Debbie Star Crunch
Little Debbie Swiss Rolls
Little Debbie Zebra Cakes
Lofthouse Sugar Cookies
Lotus Biscoff Cookies
M&Ms
Mars Twix Caramel Cookie Bars
Marshmallow Fluff

McVitie's Milk Chocolate Digestives
Mrs. Fields Chocolate Chip Cookies
Nabisco 100% Whole Grain Fig Newtons
Nabisco Barnum's Animal Crackers
Nabisco Cheese Nips
Nabisco Chips Ahoy! Cookies, Original
Nabisco Ginger Snaps
Nabisco Honey Maid Chocolate Graham
Crackers
Nabisco Honey Maid Cinnamon Graham
Crackers
Nabisco Mallomar Cookies
Nabisco Nilla Wafers
Nabisco Nutter Butter Peanut Butter
Sandwich Cookies
Nabisco Oreo Sandwich Cookies, Chocolate
Nabisco Oreo Sandwich Cookies, Golden
Nabisco Oreo Sandwich Cookies, Golden
Chocolate Creme
Nabisco Original Fig Newtons
Nabisco Premium Soup & Oyster Crackers
Nabisco Ritz Bits Cheese Sandwich Crackers
Nabisco Ritz Bits Peanut Butter Cracker
Sandwiches
Nabisco Ritz Crackers, Original
Nabisco Strawberry Newtons
Nabisco Wheat Thins, Original
Nature Valley Crunchy Granola Bars, Apple
Crisp
Nature Valley Crunchy Granola Bars, Oats 'n
Honey
Nestlé 100 Grand Chocolate Bars
Nestlé Crunch Bars
Norpro Cream Canoe Pan
Nutella
Pepperidge Farm Goldfish Baked Snack
Crackers, Cheddar
Pepperidge Farm Homestyle Sugar Cookies
Pepperidge Farm Mint Milano Cookies
Pepperidge Farm Sausalito Milk Chocolate
Macadamia Cookies
Pepperidge Farm Soft Baked Snickerdoodle
Cookies

Perfect Pan for Snow Balls
Quaker Breakfast Cookies, Oatmeal
Chocolate Chip
Quaker Breakfast Cookies, Oatmeal Raisin
Quaker Chewy Granola Bars, Oatmeal Raisin
Quaker Chewy Granola Bars, Chocolate Chip
Quaker Instant Oatmeal, Cinnamon & Spice
Quaker Instant Oatmeal, Strawberries &
Cream
Quaker Oatmeal to Go
Quaker Oatmeal to Go Brown Sugar
Cinnamon
Reese's Peanut Butter Cup
Samoas Girl Scout Cookies (a.k.a. Caramel
deLites)
Savannah Smiles Girl Scout Cookies
Sixlets
Snyder's of Hanover Pretzel Rods
Splenda No Calorie Sweetener
Splenda Sugar Blend
Sunshine Cheez-Its
Swerve
Tagalongs Girl Scout Cookies (a.k.a. Peanut
Butter Patties)
Tastykake Butterscotch Krimpets
Tastykake Peanut Butter Kandy Kakes
Thanks-A-Lot Girl Scout Cookies
Thin Mints Girl Scout Cookies
Truvia Baking Blend
USA Pans Mini Round Cake Panel Pan
Vitalicious VitaMuffin VitaTops, Banana
Chocolate Chip
Vitalicious VitaMuffin VitaTops, Blueberry
Vitalicious VitaMuffin VitaTops, Chocolate
Chip
Vitalicious VitaMuffin VitaTops, Deep
Chocolate
Weight Watchers Chocolate Brownies
Weight Watchers Chocolate Crème Cakes
Weight Watchers Lemon Crème Cakes
Whoppers Original Malted Milk Balls
Wilton 12-Cavity Spool Cake Pan
Wilton Delectovals cake pan

Acknowledgments

This book, the ones that came before it and any that may come after it, are because of my husband, Brian. His unwavering belief not only in my ability to develop 100 stellar recipes around a theme, but that you will love those recipes and tell all your friends about them—is limitless. Thank you, Brian.

Thank you to my children, Bailey, Jonathan, and Ava, for not only your insatiable appetites, but for understanding that it might look like fun, but it's still work!

To my agent, Brandi Bowles, who always gets the job done with even resolve and a stiff upper lip. I've said it before and I'll say it again: If Brandi can't get it done, it simply can't be done. Period.

To my editor, Renée Sedliar. You know when to push and when to wait things out. Your line edits are the stuff of legends, and your big-picture perspective is something I truly cherish. Plus, we speak each other's unspoken language. To Claire Ivett, whose fresh outlook and can-do attitude I have come to rely upon.

To Kate Burke, Kevin Hanover, and the rest of the marketing and publicity departments at Da Capo Press, for keeping my books on your agenda both before and after their assigned time, and doing everything you can to get them out into the world.

To Allyson Acker, my freelance publicist, for always seeing both the forest and the trees. Always the professional, I am grateful to be in your capable hands.

To Jennifer May of Jennifer May Photography. Seeing this book through your artist's eye, and then watching you bring it to life, was an honor and a thrill. You hit the right note, somewhere between whimsy and artistry, in every shot, every time. www.jennifermay.com.

To Erin Jeanne McDowell, the food stylist who was the left hand to Jennifer May's right. Erin, just as I asked, you gave me a schedule, told me how to prepare for it, and always kept us on task. I learned so much about food styling watching you work, and those lessons serve me well every day on my blog. Plus, you have truly mastered the art of the beautiful bite! www.erinjeannemcdowell.com

To Amber Morris and the rest of the production team at Perseus Books, thank you not only for being the very best at what you do, but for handling changing circumstances with aplomb.

To Alex Camlin and the rest of the design team, thank you for another beautiful cookbook. From the perfect cover all the way to the last page of the interior, everything is just as it should be.

And last but certainly not least—to my blog readers. You visit me every day, you cook and bake with me, and you buy my books—and then tell everyone from your family and friends to shoppers at the grocery store to do the same. It's clear that we're in this together, and I couldn't be more grateful.

Index

About the Author

Nicole Hunn is the personality behind the popular *Gluten-Free on a Shoestring* blog and book series. She has been featured in high-profile national print and broadcast outlets, including the *New York Times, Parade* magazine, *Better Homes and Gardens, Parents* magazine, Epicurious.com, ABC News, *The Better Show,* Sirius/XM Radio, and many others. Nicole has also been a contributing gluten-free expert for SheKnows.com Food and *Living Without* and *Gluten-Free Living* magazines. She lives in Westchester County, New York, with her husband and children. For more information and recipes, please visit www.glutenfreeonashoestring.com.